Positive CBT

Positive CBT

Individual and Group Treatment Protocols for Positive Cognitive Behavioral Therapy

Fredrike Bannink

Nicole Geschwind

hogrefe

Library of Congress of Congress Cataloging in Publication information for the print version of this book is available via the Library of Congress Marc Database under the Library of Congress Control Number 2020952417

Library and Archives Canada Cataloguing in Publication

Title: Positive CBT : individual and group treatment protocols for positive cognitive behavioral therapy / Fredrike Bannink, Nicole Geschwind.
Names: Bannink, Fredrike, author. | Geschwind, Nicole, author.
Description: Includes bibliographical references.
Identifiers: Canadiana (print) 20210095202 | Canadiana (ebook) 20210095261 | ISBN 9780889375789 (softcover) | ISBN 9781616765781 (PDF) | ISBN 9781613345788 (EPUB)
Subjects: LCSH: Cognitive therapy. | LCSH: Positive psychology.
Classification: LCC RC489.C63 B36 2021 | DDC 616.89/1425—dc23

www.hogrefe.com

PUBLISHING OFFICES

USA:	Hogrefe Publishing Corporation, 361 Newbury Street, 5th Floor, Boston, MA 02115 Phone (857) 880-2002; E-mail customerservice@hogrefe.com
EUROPE:	Hogrefe Publishing GmbH, Merkelstr. 3, 37085 Göttingen, Germany Phone +49 551 99950-0, Fax +49 551 99950-111; E-mail publishing@hogrefe.com

SALES & DISTRIBUTION

USA:	Hogrefe Publishing, Customer Services Department, 30 Amberwood Parkway, Ashland, OH 44805 Phone (800) 228-3749, Fax (419) 281-6883; E-mail customerservice@hogrefe.com
UK:	Hogrefe Publishing, c/o Marston Book Services Ltd., 160 Eastern Ave., Milton Park, Abingdon, OX14 4SB, UK Phone +44 1235 465577, Fax +44 1235 465556; E-mail direct.orders@marston.co.uk
EUROPE:	Hogrefe Publishing, Merkelstr. 3, 37085 Göttingen, Germany Phone +49 551 99950-0, Fax +49 551 99950-111; E-mail publishing@hogrefe.com

OTHER OFFICES

CANADA:	Hogrefe Publishing Corporation, 82 Laird Drive, East York, Ontario M4G 3V1
SWITZERLAND:	Hogrefe Publishing, Länggass-Strasse 76, CH-3000 Bern 9

Printed and bound in the USA

ISBN 978-0-88937-578-9 (print) · ISBN 978-1-61676-578-1 (PDF) · ISBN 978-1-61334-578-8 (EPUB)
http://doi.org/10.1027/00578-000

Preface

Life can only be understood backwards, but it must be lived forwards.

Søren Kierkegaard, Danish philosopher

Positive cognitive behavioral therapy (positive CBT) does not focus on what is wrong with our clients and how to repair that, but on what goes well in their lives and how to build on that. The focus is on the person, not the disease; the well-being of our clients takes center stage. And it does not only concern the well-being of our clients, but also our own well-being as cognitive behavioral therapists.

Positive CBT is not only an important different perspective for clients, but also for ourselves as therapists, as an antidote to burnout and negativity.

Prof. Filip Raes, Belgium
Source: Positieve cognitieve gedragstherapie
© 2014 Fredrike Bannink

Practicing Positive CBT integrates the research and practice of positive psychology and solution-focused brief therapy within the cognitive behavioral therapeutic framework. Bannink's book Practicing Positive CBT, which was published in 2012, describes her model of positive CBT and is the founding text in positive CBT. This form of CBT, also called fourth wave CBT, is now practiced worldwide, from Japan to Brazil and from Germany to Iran, and is being applied with various diagnoses. The book on this subject by Fredrike Bannink has so far been translated into Dutch, German, Japanese, Farsi, and Portuguese, and there is interest in more translations.

Fredrike Bannink captures the essential importance of building on positive feelings, motives, imagery, memories, and behaviors. The psychology of "cultivation," so much a focus in Buddhist approaches to human suffering, is brought to life in new ways with extensive knowledge of the research literature. Full of fascinating insights and practical applications, this is a book to change what we focus on and how we do work in helping people change. A book to read many times.

Prof. Paul Gilbert, UK
Source: Practicing Positive CBT: From Reducing Distress to Building Success.
© 2012 Fredrike Bannink

In recent years we have received many requests to provide a treatment protocol for positive CBT. Many colleagues have asked us to provide a "cookbook," a manual, to enable them to apply positive CBT in their workplace. We are happy to be able to offer two protocols now: a protocol for individual positive CBT and a protocol for positive CBT in a group (see Chapter 3 and Chapter 4). The protocol for individual positive CBT in the treatment of major depressive disorders has been studied at Maastricht University, the Netherlands, by Nicole Geschwind and colleagues. Nicole actually obtained her PhD at Maastricht University, researching the value of positive emotion in the treatment of depression (Geschwind, 2011).

The individual positive CBT protocol in the treatment of major depressive disorders showed promising results in that study. Moreover, clients preferred positive CBT over traditional CBT, as is evident from the quotes we have included from the study throughout this book. We describe our quantitative and qualitative research in more detail in Chapter 2. Articles describing the complete study were published in *Behavior Research and Therapy* and in *Psychotherapy* (Geschwind et al., 2019, 2020).

Now I am really building the life that I want.
Client

You will find a detailed description of the protocol for positive CBT in a group in eight sessions in Chapter 4. Fredrike developed this protocol in collaboration with her colleague Fourough Jafari from the Azad University of Tehran.

In Chapter 5 we describe Carin's case, in the hope of providing a concrete picture of what positive CBT can look like. Chapter 6 lists 12 frequently asked questions and our answers. We provide answers to questions such as, "What if my client cannot find a goal?" and "Isn't positive CBT a bit problem-phobic?"

The two Appendices contain the client's Workbooks: one for individual positive CBT and one for positive CBT in a group. As a purchaser of this book, you may use the Workbooks and exercises for your clinical work, as long as you give credit to the source.

We prefer to call the first and second wave in CBT "traditional" instead of "negative," as some colleagues have suggested. It is also our preference to speak of "clients" instead of "patients," because we believe this latter term tends to invite passivity.

To use the positive CBT protocols properly, please take note of the following:

- It is recommended that you read the entire protocol before you start the sessions with your client or group. It would also be helpful to read the description of the exercise and the associated homework suggestions before each session, as well to take a look at the clients' Workbook.
- The two client's Workbooks can be found in the Appendix 1 and Appendix 2. Therapists can download the Workbooks and their worksheets for use in the clinical work (please see the appendix on how to access these).

After having focused for almost twenty years on what is wrong with my clients, this approach feels like a breath of fresh air.
Cognitive Behavioral Therapist

We wish you lots of inspiration, and hope that positive CBT will contribute to the well-being of your clients and yourself. After all, life must be lived forwards.

Fredrike Bannink & Nicole Geschwind

Contents

Preface v

Chapter 1: Positive Cognitive Behavioral Therapy **1**
Introduction 1
Three Approaches Within Positive CBT 2
Comparing Traditional and Positive CBT 6
Comparing Traditional and Positive CBT Processes 7
Role of the Positive CBT Therapist 15

Chapter 2: Research Into Positive CBT for Depression **17**
Introduction 17
Results of the Quantitative Study 18
Results of the Qualitative Study 20
Conclusions 24

Chapter 3: Individual Positive CBT Protocol **25**
Introduction 25
Overview of the Individual Positive CBT Protocol 31
Overview of the Sessions 32
Session 1 33
Session 2 37
Session 3 41
Session 4 43
Session 5 49
Session 6 52
Session 7 56
Session 8 60

Chapter 4: Positive Cognitive Behavioral Therapy Protocol in a Group **63**
Introduction 63
Positive CBT in a Group 63
Brief Overview of Positive CBT Protocol in a Group 64
Overview of the Sessions 68
Session 1 71
Session 2 76

Session 3 81
Session 4 85
Session 5 88
Session 6 91
Session 7 95
Session 8 98
Comparison With the Protocol for Individual Therapy 101

Chapter 5: Case Carin **103**
Introduction 103
Carin 103

Chapter 6: Frequently Asked Questions **109**
Introduction 109
Twelve Frequently Asked Questions and Our Answers 109

Epilogue **116**

References **117**

Appendix: Tools and Resources **121**
Client's Workbook for Positive Cognitive Behavioral Therapy With Individuals 122
Client's Workbook for Positive CBT in a Group 130

Acknowledgments **141**

About the Authors **143**

Notes on Supplementary Materials **144**

Chapter 1
Positive Cognitive Behavioral Therapy

The secret to change is to focus all of your energy,
not on fighting the old, but on building the new.

Seneca, Roman philosopher

Introduction

Positive cognitive behavioral therapy (positive CBT) integrates the research and practice of the positive psychology movement and of solution-focused brief therapy (SFBT) within the cognitive behavioral therapeutic framework (Bannink, 2012). It is a competency-based approach that shifts the focus away from what is wrong with clients and what does not work, to what goes well and does work in their lives.

This competency-based approach – an approach that looks for existing competencies of clients – focuses on uncovering and expanding their skill repertoire. Competency implies that we have sufficient skills to adequately perform the tasks necessary in daily life. The principles of the competency-based approach are:

- Connect with the strengths of your clients and activate those strengths in helping your clients to realize their goals.
- Listen to your clients' needs, wishes, limits, and norms, and take these seriously.
- Focus on creating new opportunities.

Client:
Sometimes I feel a bit guilty. When I got up a few days ago and saw that the sun was shining I wanted to go out and have a coffee on a terrace. A little voice inside of me said I shouldn't do that, because my sister just died. When a friend phoned me and I told her that I was sitting on a terrace, she said, "What? Am I calling the right number?"

Three Approaches Within Positive CBT

In this section we briefly discuss the three approaches that come together in positive CBT: traditional CBT, positive psychology, and SFBT. We will provide a comparison of traditional and positive CBT and their processes, and discuss the different role of the positive CBT therapist in each approach. To mention just a few highlights: In positive CBT, goal formulation replaces problem exploration; a focus on competencies replaces a focus on deficits; self-monitoring is used with exceptions to the problem instead of the problem itself; the upward arrow technique is used instead of the downward arrow technique; and the focus is on behavior maintenance instead of on relapse prevention.

Cognitive Behavioral Therapy

The roots of CBT can be traced to the development of behavior therapy in the early 1920s, of cognitive therapy in the 1960s, and the subsequent merging of these two. *Cognitive therapy* assumes that maladaptive behavior and disturbed mood are the result of inappropriate or irrational thinking patterns, called *automatic thoughts*. Instead of reacting to the reality of a given situation, an individual reacts to their own distorted viewpoint of the situation. In therapy, clients are made aware of these distorted thinking patterns and change them (cognitive restructuring). *Behavioral therapy*, or behavioral modification, trains clients to replace undesirable behaviors with healthier behavioral patterns. *CBT* integrates the cognitive restructuring approach of cognitive therapy with the behavioral modification techniques of behavioral therapy. Many CBT programs have been tested for their effectiveness: The emphasis is on applying evidence-based treatments. This is the basis for CBT often being preferred over other psychotherapeutic methods.

Traditional CBT may be seen as a class of treatments which have the same features in common but also differ in important aspects. It is problem-focused and structured toward the client; it requires honesty and openness between the client and therapist, as the therapist offers strategies and asks the client to apply and evaluate them. Guided discovery or Socratic questioning is often used to help clients to gain insights.

Positive Psychology

Positive psychology was developed in the 1990s as a scientific movement that tries to understand positive human functioning – its cognitions, emotions, and behavior. It is the study of what makes life worth living and what makes people and societies thrive. The movement is focused on bringing out the best in oneself and others with the aim of functioning optimally. The focus is not only on reducing problems or complaints, but also on increasing strengths and well-being. This strengths-based approach – identifying and deploying your strengths – offers a good starting point for further conversations.

When looking at mental health, we find that health is not same as the absence of disease. Mental health concerns both the absence of pathology *as well as* the presence of well-being. Psychotherapy should therefore no longer be the place where only problems are discussed and repaired, but also the place where strengths are discovered, positive emotions are reinforced, and hope, gratitude, and optimism are nourished (Bannink & Peeters, 2020).

Research shows that psychopathology and positive mental health are two different complementary indicators of mental health (Keyes, 2005). And although psychological problems are more often associated with poor positive mental health than with good, their relationship is limited. The degree of psychopathology does not say much about the degree of positive mental health, and vice versa. Someone with serious psychiatric disorders can still experience a high degree of well-being, and the other way around – absence of mental disorders does not guarantee a high degree of well-being.

Nowadays, positive psychology has a large body of completed research examining its constructs, including optimism, well-being, gratitude, resilience, flow, hope, courage, and positive emotion. The most common theory in the positive psychology field is the well-being theory of Martin Seligman (2011). Five pillars together ensure well-being: positive emotion, engagement, positive relationships, meaning, and accomplishment, which give the acronym PERMA. The five pillars in more detail are

1. *Positive emotion:* Focusing on positive emotions is more than just smiling; it is the ability to be optimistic and view the past, present, and future from a positive perspective. This positive view of life, where there is room for fun and enjoyment, can help us in relationships and work, and inspire us to be more creative and take more chances. It is about experiencing positive emotions: To what extent do we feel happy and content?
2. *Engagement:* Finding activities that take our full engagement helps us to learn, grow, and nurture personal happiness. This life of involvement refers to our commitment to do what we do: To what extent do we experience a sense of personal fulfillment?
3. *Relationships:* Having relationships and social connections is one of the most important aspects of life. We are social animals that thrive on connection, love, intimacy, and a strong emotional and physical interaction with other humans. Building positive relationships with our parents, siblings, peers, and friends is important for spreading love and joy. Having strong relationships gives us support in difficult times.
4. *Meaning:* Finding meaning and a reason we are on this earth is important to living a life of happiness and fulfillment. Rather than the pursuit of pleasure and material wealth, there is an actual purpose for our life. To understand the greater impact of our work and why we choose to pursue that work will help us enjoy our tasks more and become more satisfied and happier. Living a meaningful life is not only about us, but also about something larger than us – about altruism and caring for others: To what extent do we have the feeling of being part of, and contributing to, a greater whole?
5. *Accomplishment:* Having goals and ambition in life is important also. We should make realistic goals that can be met; just putting in the effort to achieve those goals can already give us a sense of satisfaction. When we finally achieve them, we will experience a sense of pride and fulfillment. Pursuing success, accomplishment, winning, achievement, and mastery for their own sake will help us thrive and flourish.

The higher you score on all five pillars – the higher the sum – the greater your well-being is (Bannink, 2017a). Well-being is important because it forms an important buffer against psychopathology. Recently there seems to be a growing consent to choose the letter V for Vitality as the sixth building block of well-being. Vitality is about taking good care of our body and mind – for example, by exercising regularly, following a healthy diet, getting enough sleep, and applying mindfulness. Seligman, cofounder of the positive psychology movement, states

> The message of the positive psychology movement is to remind our field that it has been deformed. Psychology is not just the study of disease, weakness, and damage; it is also the study of strength and virtue. Treatment is not just fixing what is wrong; it is also building what is right. (Seligman, 2005, p. 4)

Client:
At the request of my therapist I asked a few friends to write down my strenghts and virtues. Scary, but at the same time fun. They wrote that I was someone they can rely on, I tend to forget that sometimes. So I thought: if they think they can rely on me, then I may well see myself in the same way.

Tayyab Rashid (2009) mentions four implications that positive psychotherapy has:

1. *Positive psychology interventions* (PPIs) do not imply that other interventions are negative.
2. People quickly get used to new circumstances. To experience more well-being, people must regularly develop new activities that fit with their values, strengths, and interests.
3. It is intended that PPIs invite people to consider new activities and not prescribe them what to do. Attention must also be paid to individual and cultural differences with regard to happiness and well-being.
4. PPIs are not only intended for people with problems or disorders; positive psychology also relates to work, education, insight, love, growth, and play.

Client:
My psychologist said: "You can compare your body with a car. If you only look at defects and everything that is wrong or may go wrong, you no longer enjoy driving. And that is exactly what I want you to have: a nice ride. Therefore, I want us to discover how you can enjoy driving.

Solution-Focused Brief Therapy

In SFBT, building solutions is central, not solving or reducing problems. It consists of the pragmatic application of a number of principles and exercises, best described as finding the direct route to what works (De Shazer, 1985, 1991; Bannink, 2010, 2015b).

The two solution-focused simple assumptions are:

1. If something works (better), do more of it.
2. If something does not work, stop and do something else.

SFBT is a structured process, with ample acknowledgment for the suffering that the problems or complaints cause. However, problems need not to be analyzed. There is a useful interaction with the therapist in which clients find solutions and are invited to change. By focusing on what works in their lives, they gain more hope, have more creative ideas, feel more competent, and see more possibilities.

SFBT helps clients to develop a vision of a better future and to take notice of – both by the client and the therapist – their strengths and resources. Clients may then apply those to make their vision a reality.

Solution-focused questions lie at the heart of SFBT: They invite clients to think differently, notice positive differences, and achieve desired changes. SFBT does not work on the basis of systematically investigated or general applications, as positive psychology does. It is all about finding what works for this client, at this moment, in this context. The techniques and specific solution-focused questions have been researched by Franklin et al. (2012).

The solution-focused approach is complementary to the medical model. The approach is about starting or expanding desired behavior. It is goal- and future-oriented, short and practical, and focuses on concrete results. It is light and positive in tone, and it saves energy at the end of the day. Some solution-focused assumptions include

- You do not need to know the cause or perpetuating factors of a complaint or problem to resolve it.
- A quick change or solution of the problem is possible.
- Focus on solutions and possibilities instead of on pathology.
- Invite clients to take action.
- Look, together with the client, for small positive changes, and amplify those.

Client:
I wanted to resume my life after my wife's death and meet new people. First I wanted to write a letter to apply to volunteer at the library, but it just didn't happen. My GP asked me: "How are you going to write that letter? How will you start? Where will you be sitting?" I replied that I would be sitting at my table with my laptop. We discussed a few more details, and then my GP asked me: "When will you come and tell me that you succeeded?" "Next Friday," I said. "I now work in the library for three mornings a week and enjoy it."

In SFBT, the role of therapists is different from other forms of psychotherapy: They are no longer the only experts who make the diagnoses and give advice, but they consider their clients to be coexperts in the field of their own lives. Research shows that SFBT usually requires fewer sessions than problem-focused psychotherapy, and therefore SFBT is more cost-effective. Research also shows that the clients' autonomy is well guaranteed, and there is less burnout among practitioners (Franklin et al., 2012; Medina & Beyebach, 2014). SFBT cofounder Insoo Kim Berg, a few months before she passed away, wrote in her Foreword for Fredrike Bannink's Dutch book *Oplossingsgerichte vragen. Handboek oplossingsgerichte gespreksvoering*, 4th ed. (Bannink, 2019, first published in 2006), which was later published in English as *1001 Solution-Focused Questions. Handbook for Solution-Focused Interviewing*:

> Solution-focused interviewing is based on the respectful assumption that clients have the inner resources to construct highly individualized and uniquely effective solutions to their problems. (Bannink, 2010, p. xi)

Client:
If I had had a suicide pill, I am not sure I would not have taken it. I thought: "I'll never be able to get out of this." My therapist then asked me why I would not have taken that pill. And then I thought of all the things in my life that I find important, the lovely people that I know, my hobbies and vacations. And then the sun started to shine again.

> Client:
> My therapist told me that you don't always have to know the cause of a problem to be able to start working on improvement[s] by taking small steps. And that you can start searching for possibilities and the beginning of success, rather than dwell on the impossibilities. I then told her that I had recently started a mindfulness training [sic], hoping it will help me to become a bit more relaxed. She thought that was a good example of what works for me. And that I can start looking for more things that work or have worked for me. I then suggested continuing to work with the mindfulness trainer because I had already spoken with him. My therapist said she thought this was a very good idea.

Comparing Traditional and Positive CBT

As we wrote earlier, CBT can be seen as a class of treatments, with some similarities and some differences among them. The purpose of all forms of CBT is to help clients to make desired changes in their lives.

When we look at positive CBT, it differs from traditional CBT in two important aspects:

1. Traditional CBT has an explicit theory about the cause and/or perpetuating factors of problems. SFBT has no assumptions about how people end up in difficulties. Steve De Shazer, cofounder of SFBT, once summarized this rather bluntly: "Shit happens." Positive CBT assumes that well-being can be increased by focusing on the positive things in life (see PERMA; Seligman, 2011).
2. Traditional CBT assumes that knowledge about the cause or perpetuating factors in problems is necessary to help clients get better. Positive CBT assumes that the (causes or perpetuating factors in) problems do not tell us how we as therapists can be useful for our clients.

We see positive CBT as fourth wave CBT. It is future-focused and offers hope for a better life. It is about designing an outcome that was not there before. Positive CBT is transdiagnostic – it can be applied to all mental disorders – and is also transcultural. Currently positive CBT is used worldwide, from Japan to Brazil and from Germany to Iran.

Fredrike Bannink described the learning theory implications and further theoretical points of view in her book *Practicing Positive CBT* (Bannink, 2012). She also described what already can be seen as more positive within traditional CBT. Third wave CBT can be thought of in terms of approaches such as competitive memory training (COMET), acceptance and commitment therapy (ACT; Hayes et al., 2003), and behavior activation (Ferster, 1973; Beck, 2011).

> Client:
> People should pay more attention to everything that goes well, and that is exactly what this therapy is about. I noticed that if I pick out the things that do go well, the things that do not go well naturally become less important.

Client:
I now feel a much stronger woman. What I realize is that I am linked with this society and that I do matter. That is a big difference compared to the situation before this therapy. I have had psychotherapy for many years focusing on my traumas.

Client:
At first I thought: traditional psychotherapy will probably be more helpful. But in the end my thoughts about traditional CBT were: if I have more of these sessions, I'll quit. With positive CBT I was reluctant at first, I thought that won't work, but I have learned ten times more from it. You really start to look at yourself differently and apply things much better. It is a steeper path, but it is much better. For me, positive CBT was a turning point, because I really enjoyed going to the sessions and thought: this is gonna help me.

Comparing Traditional and Positive CBT Processes

The CBT process has three general phases: diagnosis, treatment, and closing phase. Then, in traditional CBT, we see the following more specific phases: problem exploration, choosing a problem to work on, self-monitoring of the problem, designing functional behavioral analyses, specifying a plan and objectives, applying modification procedures, and evaluation during the closing of the therapy.

The phases in traditional CBT versus positive CBT processes are shown in Figure 1 and highlighted in the following paragraphs. You may notice that positive CBT has one phase fewer than traditional CBT.

The *first phase*, introduction and building rapport is more or less the same in positive CBT as it is in traditional CBT. One difference is that from the start of the session, the focus in positive CBT is positive: What does the client do in daily life? What do they think they are doing well? What do they like about the things they are doing? Also, the therapist asks about any *pretreatment change* since the client first contacted the therapist. A significant number of clients will already be able to mention positive changes when they come for the first session (Weiner-Davis et al., 1987). To find out what these changes are, the therapist should, of course, ask that particular question.

The *second phase* in positive CBT concerns the goal formulation (instead of the problem exploration in traditional CBT): It is about designing an outcome that was not there before (using the *synthesis paradigm*, which is looking forward to what might be created, instead of the *analysis paradigm*, which is looking back at what already is). The therapist invites the client to provide a detailed description of their preferred future. In traditional CBT, attention to a plan and objectives is only given in the fifth phase, when the overall diagnostic phase has been finished. In traditional CBT, therapists usually pay no explicit attention to the collaborative relationship that the therapist has with the client. This concerns questions such as, "To what extent is the client motivated to change?" "Who will do what to achieve this change, and when?" Positive CBT is not about goals or objectives (plural); there is just one goal, this being the preferred future or outcome of the client (and of important others

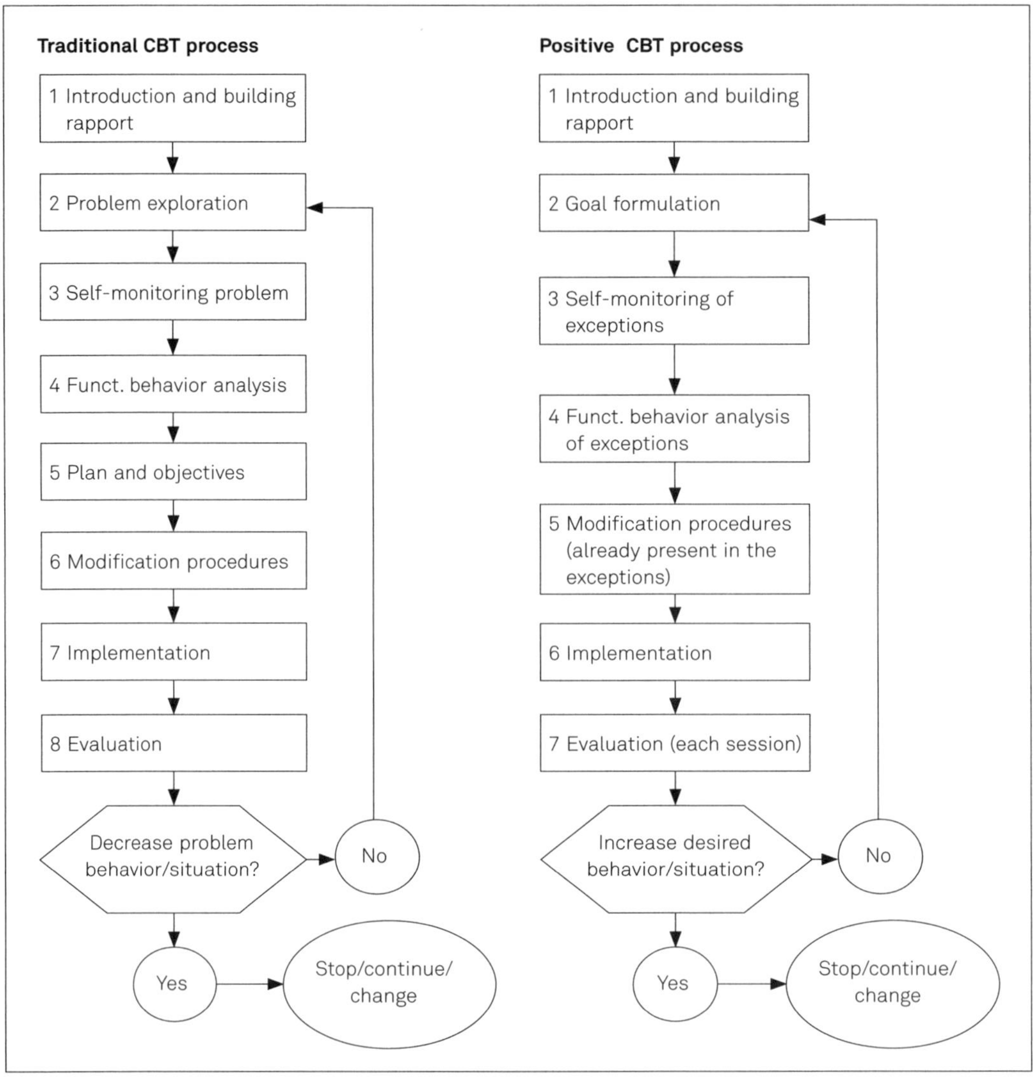

Figure 1 Comparing the traditional and positive CBT processes.

in their life), with a focus on desired behavior, desired cognitions, and desired emotions. This goal is stated in positive, achievable, and concrete terms.

Objectives (plural) in traditional CBT are usually formulated in negative terms, such as "to worry less" or "to decrease depression." This is also seen in book titles that are based on traditional CBT: *How to overcome your fear*, *Help yourself get out of depression*, and *How to deal with trauma*.

It may be useful for your clients to make the following comparison: "Before you go to the supermarket, do you sometimes make a shopping list?" If the client answers affirmatively, then ask, "Do you put things on that list that you do NOT want to buy? It would become a very long list, because in the supermarket you can actually buy around 5,000 things... Of course not! You'll make a list of what you DO want to buy."

So, while traditional CBT focuses on goals or objectives (plural), in positive CBT, the question is always: "Suppose you have reached your goal, what will your new and better life look like?" For example, if one of the goals of the client is to become more assertive, the therapist might ask, "So suppose you become as assertive as you want to be, how will your life be different from what it is now? What will you think, feel, and do differently?" The therapist thus asks questions about all of the positive differences the client can come up with. Working on objectives (plural) has the risk that if an objective such as becoming more assertive is not achieved, the therapy may get stuck, and the client's preferred future does not come closer, or it may even disappear from view. There are always more roads (goals or subgoals) to Rome (being the preferred future or outcome). As they say: All roads lead to Rome! If one road is not possible, then the client and therapist can look for another road. And just to be clear: It is the client who decides what the goal should look like, not the therapist.

Questions about goal formulation in positive CBT include, "What will be the best outcome for you from this therapy?" or "How will we know you no longer need to come here?" or, in the case of n mandated (involuntary) client, "When will the person or institute who referred you think you no longer need to come here?" Or you may ask, "What are your best hopes?" "And what difference will it make for you and/or for important others when everything you hope for has become a reality?" or "What will your new and better life look like?" Or you may ask, "When does this therapy or this session get an 8 (or a 9, or even a 10)?"

Client:
I don't want to be on the edge every time and fear that my depression is coming back again. I want to take 10 steps in the right direction. I don't want to think: I hope I don't turn 40. I want to think that life is worth living and hope I can make it worthwhile. So, what are my best hopes? That I won't be depressed 90% of the time in a year's time, but only 50%. That it has become a habit to see the beautiful and good little things in life.

Sometimes people ask whether positive CBT might be a bit *problem-phobic*, but this is not the case. Clients get the opportunity to describe briefly what is going on in their lives (see also Chapter 6). The difference with traditional CBT is that the therapist does not ask questions about the details of the problem (and thus does not reinforce the client's *problem talk*). However, the therapist does give acknowledgment to the difficult situations client find themselves in, asking, for example, "Am I correct in understanding that this must be a very tough situation for you?"

Positive CBT does not use the phase of problem exploration and problem selection, as is common in traditional CBT. It uses the method of *stepped diagnosis* (Bakker et al., 2010): In the first and second echelons of mental health, the treatment can start right away; but only if the necessary diagnostics are added.

Constructing a holistic therory about the causal relationships between problems, as is often done in traditional CBT, is not necessary in positive CBT. Searching for causes and/ or perpetuating factors usually only leads to statements, most likely not to solutions. Also, searching for explanatory assumptions is seen as superfluous.

Client:
And then my psychiatrist asked, "What do you want?" I was surprised: I was never asked this question in the many admissions I had. The question in itself is not difficult, but if no one ever askes you, you have to think about it for a while.

I thought: Yes, what do I actually want? I don't want to feel so depressed anymore that I don't want to live. I know these thoughts will always be there. But I want life to be bearable. And then we could start talking about what a bearable life looks like for me. And we could talk about when glimpses of it were already visible.

The *third phase* of both traditional and positive CBT processes is self-monitoring. In positive CBT, self-monitoring is not done with regard to the intensity and/or frequency of the problem, as is done in traditional CBT, but with regard to the exceptions to the problem. The therapist asks about the times when the problem or complaint could have been there, but for some reason was not (or was less). There are always fluctuations; nothing stays the same. The ancient Greeks referred to this with the phrase *panta rhei* (everything flows). It is therefore not a question of *if* there are or have been exceptions, but *when* there are or were there exceptions. Asking for exceptions is important in any psychotherapy, because finding exceptions may influence a differential diagnosis. If, for example, a child cannot sit still at home but can sit still in the classroom (an exception to the problem), then attention-deficit/ hyperactivity disorder cannot be diagnosed.

The questions to find exceptions are:

- When is/was the problem not there, or is/was less (even if only a little bit)?
- When is/was the problem (temporarily) not a problem?
- When is/was there a glimpse of what you want to have instead of the problem (the preferred future or outcome)?
- When is/was the problem there, but you can/could cope with it (a little bit) better?

In the exceptions, we find the solutions and competencies of our clients. So the solutions do not have to come from the therapist! This ensures the therapist can feel less responsible for giving advice and being the only expert in the room. In positive CBT, clients are seen as coexperts!

> For the client, the problem is seen as primary (and exceptions, if seen at all, are seen as secondary). For therapists, the exceptions are seen as primary; interventions are meant to help clients make a similar inversion, which will lead to the development of a solution. (De Shazer, 1991, p. 58; cofounder of SFBT)

It is important to have an eye for what works in the client's life and for what they have achieved, because these positive expectations ensure that further improvement is possible. Even in the toughest circumstances, there are still things that go well (enough). Therefore, during the entire positive CBT, clients keep track of these exceptions and write them down in their Diary of Better Moments. They also write what they did differently to make these exceptions happen.

Client:
I said, "I always feel bad," and then my therapist said, "No one is feeling bad 24/7. Even if you don't notice, there are always a few seconds when you smile, or when things are not too bad. You don't have to be completely happy, but there are always times when things are not that bad." First I thought: Oh no, not for me. And then I started paying attention to those moments, and I thought: Oh yes, it's true. Those moments are there after all. And these were not the big things, for example, my kitten, that looked at me so sweetly. I thought: I can see this. And then I knew I could start seeing these things more often.

In the *fourth phase* of both traditional and positive CBT processes – based on the self-monitoring of exceptions, in the case of positive CBT – the therapist and client may make positive functional behavior analyses together, using the same *antecedent, behavior, consequence model* (ABC model) that is used in traditional CBT. It is possible to have the procedure started at the desired behavior (which may not be shown or not be shown enough). Only the therapeutic measures should then be mirrored. Inhibitory "C"s (consequences) should be undermined, and stimulating "C"s should be strengthened.

The *fifth phase* of positive CBT is the modification procedures; the *sixth phase* is its implementation (in traditional CBT, these are the sixth and seventh phases). The modification procedures in positive CBT do not have to be suggested by the therapist, but are based on what works in the client's life. They can be found by finding exceptions. The following solution-focused assumptions apply: If something works, do more of it; if something is not working, stop and do something else.

The therapist invites clients to talk about their strengths, competencies, and resources. These are then used to solve the problem or complaint and bring the preferred future closer. Clients are invited to talk about their strengths or complete the Values in Action (VIA) Character Strengths Survey (https://www.viacharacter.org/). That questionnaire has been developed as a classification system of 6 values and 24 strengths, as a counterpart to the classification system of the *Diagnostic and Statistical Manual of Mental Disorders,* 5th edition (DSM-5; Peterson, 2006).

Behavioral therapists Kuyken and colleagues comment on finding and deploying strengths during the case conceptualization and during the further course of treatment in the following terms:

> We advocate for therapists to identify and work with client strengths at every stage or case conceptualization. A strengths' focus is often more engaging for clients and offers the advantages of harnessing clients' strengths in the change process to pave a way to lasting recovery. (Kuyken et al., 2009, p. 28)

In addition to looking at strengths and resources, positive CBT also looks at helpful cognitions and beliefs, and helpful behavior. This is not done by developing and testing new cognitions, beliefs, and behaviors, but by finding and expanding positive cognitions, beliefs, and behavior that every client already possesses – at least to a certain extent. Dysfunctional cognitions need not be found and challenged (in any quest to repair what is wrong).

Whereas in traditional CBT, the therapist challenges dysfunctional cognitions using the *downward arrow technique* to detect core beliefs that cause negative client reactions to certain situations, positive CBT uses the *upward arrow technique*. With this approach, clients detect beliefs that cause positive responses to certain situations. The question is not: "What is the worst that can happen?" but "What is the best that can happen?" It is about the best-case scenario instead of the worst-case scenario.

In positive CBT, the therapist does not have to find and supply the modification procedures; they are already available to clients, and they have used them before successfully. This increases the chance that they will apply them again, compared with cases in which the therapist is giving advice or suggestions.

In sum: in the exceptions, we find the clients' competencies and all of the things that work (in their lives). From a solution-focused perspective, the suggestion is, if something works (better), do more of it!

> Client:
> I became more aware of all the good things around me during therapy. And I became aware that I have a lot of influence on what happens. My way of thinking influences the things that happen around me or happen to me. That is what I like about this therapy, this realization.

> Client:
> What I like about this approach is that my psychologist says: You have actually already conquered many things. It is great that you go to work again, meet your friends, and you permit your family to reassure you. How did you manage to do all that? She just shows me: You already do many things right.

Scaling questions invite clients to put their observations, impressions, and predictions on a scale from 10 to 0. For example, "On a scale of 10 to 0, where 10 means the ideal situation, and 0 the opposite, where do you want to be? What is a realistic goal?" Or, "How exactly does your situation look at that number?" The follow-up question is, "What number do you give to your current situation on that scale? How is it, that it's not lower? What else is there in that number? And what else?"

The therapist then works with the client on further progression. Questions that can be posed include, "What will be the next signs of progress? How will you or important others notice that the situation is a little better?" or "What little step can you take to get closer to your goal?" "What does a number higher on the scale look like?" and "Who or what may be useful to help you get there?" It is not the big steps, but the small, feasible ones that lead to major changes. We call them the "baby steps." What can the client do today, tomorrow, or the day after tomorrow? In addition to the topic of progress, scaling questions can be about the motivation, hope, or confidence that clients have that they will reach their goal.

Positive CBT considers doing *homework* to be less important than traditional CBT does: In positive CBT, change of perspective often already takes place during the session. Only if clients find it useful, the therapist may give some homework suggestions. We prefer to use terms such as "suggestions" rather than "tasks" or "assignments," because for many people, these last terms have a negative connotation. The therapist is flexible when it comes to making homework suggestions. If the client does not want or has not done a homework suggestion, they must surely have a good reason. The therapist will then ask for more details about their good reasons. If the client wants to do the homework in a different way, or continue longer than the protocol indicates, that is fine too.

The homework suggestions are either observation suggestions or behavior suggestions, depending on the collaborative relationship between the therapist and the client. The extent of a collaborative relationship has already been evaluated during the first session: Is the client mandated and do they come involuntarily (we call this a *visitor relationship*)? Does the client think that someone else or something else should change (we call this a *complainant relationship*). Or is this a client who is motivated to change (we call this a *customer relationship*). Please note: these relationship labels always concern the collaborative relationship between therapist and client and are not an individual characteristic of each client. If a customer relationship does not yet exist, it is up to the therapist to invite clients to change (that should be part of the therapist's expertise) and thereby change the collaborative relationship with their client into a customer relationship.

Clients with whom the therapist has a visitor relationship (involuntary clients) receive no homework suggestions. After all, they do not have a problem themselves, but come to see a therapist because a referrer has asked them to do so (think of a partner, parents, school, supervisor, or probation officer). Observation suggestions are suitable for clients who do experience a problem themselves, but who do not see themselves as part of the problem and/or the solution (clients with whom the therapist has a complainant relationship). Observation suggestions include: "Notice the better moments (positive differences) and write them down in a Journal of Better Moments." Or "Observe what happens in your life that you want to keep happening, or that you do not want to change."

Behavior suggestions are only suitable for clients who do see themselves as part of the problem and/or the solution (i.e., clients with whom the therapist has a customer relationship). These include, for example, behavioral experiments in which the client manipulates the environment or makes discoveries, but always with a positive focus. This is different from traditional CBT, where clients may be asked, "Try to answer the question: 'Will people reject you when you go to that party?'" In positive CBT, clients are invited to use a more positive focus, "Find an answer to the question: 'Will people accept you when you go to that party?'" We all know that what you focus on expands!

> Client:
> My therapist asked me to write down 10 positive things about myself. That was quite difficult. I could find just a few things and that was it. Then I had to ask other people: how they see me, and what do they think are my strong points? But actually it was quite nice, because I found out that I have more strengths than I previously thought I had.

> Client:
> Writing down positive things really stayed with me, because in the beginning it was very difficult to find anything at all. In the beginning I thought, you cannot write that you have gotten out of bed. But finally I thought, that is also positive. You went outside, you called a few friends that you did not speak with for years. Those are all positive things. I never thought about it this way and didn't want to see these simple things as positive. But they are! Especially if you are depressed, such small things cost so much effort that you don't even have room for other, larger things. I mean, emotionally heavy things about which you could say something positive, which is normal for other people. So you need to the keep the bar quite low, see where you are now and live with the small positive things. That stuck with me the most.

The *seventh and final phase* is the phase of evaluation. In traditional CBT, this is the eighth phase in the process. In positive CBT, evaluation takes place at the end of each session, not only at the end of the therapy, as is sometimes done in traditional CBT. In positive CBT, the therapist asks the client for feedback, which can be done using the Session Rating Scale (SRS) or the Group Session Rating Scale (GSRS). These are feedback instruments based on the three domains that reseach has shown to be essential:

1. The collaborative relationship between therapist and client
2. Goal and topics
3. Approach or method

The therapist always asks the client what the therapist themselves could do differently or better next time, so as to get a higher rating at the end of the next session. More information about the SRS and GSRS can be found in Duncan (2010), Duncan et al. (2003), and Bannink (2012, 2014).

> Client:
> Positive CBT helped me the most. Look at the things you've done well, even if it's something small, for example, you went outside which you don't normally do, so that is something positive! Use that! Live with that! Just say, "Look, write it down, you have achieved something." It doesn't have to be big like you stopped the next world war, that is not reasonable. And you have to keep on thinking that all small things matter. That's the best I got out of positive CBT.

During *follow-up sessions*, the therapist carefully examines and evaluates together with the client what is better. The therapist asks for a detailed description of the positive exceptions, compliments the client, and puts the emphasis on the input of the client in finding these solutions.

The opening question in each follow-up session is, "What is better?" When searching for what is better, you will almost always find improvements. The implicit suggestion of this question is that something *is* going better, and that only some searching is needed to find what that may be. Experience shows that when the therapist starts every session with this question, clients will anticipate this.

From the outset of positive CBT, the therapist and client talk about its closure. Consider questions such as, "When can we stop meeting like this?" "When do you not have to come back anymore?" Or in the case of mandated clients, "When will the referrer think you no longer need to see me?" Even at the start of therapy, the client may discuss how they will celebrate when they have reached their goal (sufficiently) or have overcome the problem or complaint. Furthermore, in positive CBT, we no longer speak of *relapse prevention*, but of *behavior maintenance*. Ask your client, "What should you continue to do in order to make the chance as big as possible that these changes will last?" or "Find 50 positive changes, find 50 good reasons to hold onto those changes, and find 50 ways to do that."

With clients who have serious psychiatric disorders such as a psychosis, severe depression, or suicidal behavior, a *recovery plan* may be made. Ideas for this can be generated by asking the client about how they have regained their balance after a crisis.

Useful questions are:

- "What did you do when you felt a bit better again?"
- "How do you usually manage to come out of a depression?"

- "What have you learned from previous admissions that could be useful in the current situation?"

> Client:
> Because I have been admitted a few times because of depression I will never be able to work as a lawyer. I don't have a partner either. For a long time, I only could think about what I do not have and cannot do, but that did not bring me any further. Now together with a psychologist I look at what I do and can do which makes me much happier. I am now doing a training course in a direction of which I already dreamed as a child.

Role of the Positive CBT Therapist

The role of the positive CBT therapist differs from the role of the traditional CBT therapist. It can best be described as *not knowing*. The therapist is not the only expert in the room who gives advice, as is done in traditional psychotherapies. By describing their role as not knowing, it is meant that therapists ask open questions in a curious and inviting manner to bring out and make use of the client's expertise. In this way, clients are invited to describe their preferred future and a broad spectrum of opportunities to achieve their goal.

Positive CBT therapists see clients as experts on their own lives and let themselves be informed by them. Clients are the ones who determine how they want to design their preferred future and their solutions to get there. The therapists do not have to push or pull. Research shows that working with such a positive focus is more effective in reducing burnout among professionals than working with a negative focus (Medina & Beyebach, 2014).

> Client:
> My therapist gives me the feeling that I am not a problem case. That I have strengths and do many things well. That I can and may find solutions myself to get my life back on track. And that's very nice.

Chapter 2
Research Into Positive CBT for Depression

It is never too late to be who you might have been.

George Eliot, English writer

Introduction

Recent research (Craske et al., 2019; Dunn et al., 2019; Geschwind et al., 2010; Geschwind, 2011; Widnall et al., 2020) suggests that a stronger focus on positive emotions and on positive mental health may increase the effectiveness of cognitive behavioral therapy (CBT). Three arguments support this assertion:

First, traditional CBT focuses primarily on reducing psychological symptoms: Treatment is deemed successful when psychopathology is in remission and residual complaints are as few as possible. However, research into clients' perspectives shows that their definition of recovery from depression is broader. Clients find it important that they function just as well or better after treatment (compared with before the onset of the depression), and that they are optimistic and hopeful, enjoy life, and feel part of society (Demyttenaere et al., 2015; Zimmerman et al., 2006). This means that a mere decrease in symptoms is not enough for them. Reduction of psychopathology in itself does not automatically translate into higher well-being (Keyes, 2005), so a stronger focus on promoting positive emotions and positive mental health is necessary. According to the *broaden-and-build theory*, positive emotions contribute to both increased resilience and reduction of symptoms (Fredrickson, 2009; Garland et al., 2010).

Second, in addition, even people without psychological problems pay more attention to negative rather than positive events. This phenomenon is known as *negativity bias* (Baumeister et al., 2001). When people are depressed, this negativity bias soon gets the upper hand (Gotlib et al., 2004). Traditional CBT may inadvertently encourage this bias by asking clients to keep track of problem situations as part of their homework, thereby focusing their attention on negative events both during and outside the therapy sessions.

Third, for clients with a depressive disorder, the absence of positive feelings such as pleasure and interest (i.e., anhedonia) is one of the two main characteristics of a depressive episode. The other characteristic is a depressed mood. The results of several studies have suggested that increases in positive emotions contribute more to well-being and to prevention of, and recovery from, depression than decreases in negative emotions (Geschwind, 2011; Geschwind et al., 2010, 2011; Khazanov & Ruscio, 2016). This implies that promoting positive emotions should be one of the main pillars of treatments for depressive disorders (Craske et al., 2016; Dunn, 2012).

Positive CBT is ideally suited to stimulate positive feelings and positive mental health, thereby potentially making treatment for depression more efficient as well as more enjoyable for clients (and maybe also for therapists). The authors of this book set up a study to investigate whether this was indeed the case. Is treatment with positive CBT more efficient and more enjoyable, compared with traditional CBT?

> Client:
> In the beginning I thought: I'm feeling so low now. Am I supposed to pretend that nothing is going on and sit here talking about fun things?

A total of 49 clients diagnosed with unipolar depressive disorder participated in the study in Maastricht, The Netherlands. They had all been referred for treatment in specialist mental health care by their GPs. After clients had given permission to participate in the study, they were randomly assigned to one of the two treatments: They either started with eight individual positive CBT sessions and then continued with eight sessions of individual traditional CBT, or the other way around. So, every client participated in the same two treatment blocks and received a total of 16 sessions of treatment.

We checked whether clients experienced more improvement during positive CBT compared with traditional CBT. We asked clients to complete a number of questionnaires before the start of the treatment as well as during treatment. Clients completed these questionnaires after every fourth session. Additionally, they completed a questionnaire on depressive symptoms (the Quick Inventory of Depressive Symptoms; Rush et al., 2003) after each session. The first 12 clients also took part in an interview about how they experienced both forms of CBT.

The results involved both a quantitative study (based on questionnaires), followed by qualitative research (based on interviews). For the quantitative research, we collaborated with colleagues Arnoud Arntz and Frenk Peeters. For the qualitative research, we collaborated with colleague Emke Bosgraaf, who conducted the interviews and carried out the qualitative analysis.

Results of the Quantitative Study

The following findings emerged from the statistical analysis (Geschwind et al., 2019): In the first study phase of eight sessions, both treatments worked approximately equally well with regard to the reduction of depressive symptoms. However, in the second study phase of eight sessions, positive CBT worked significantly better than traditional CBT.

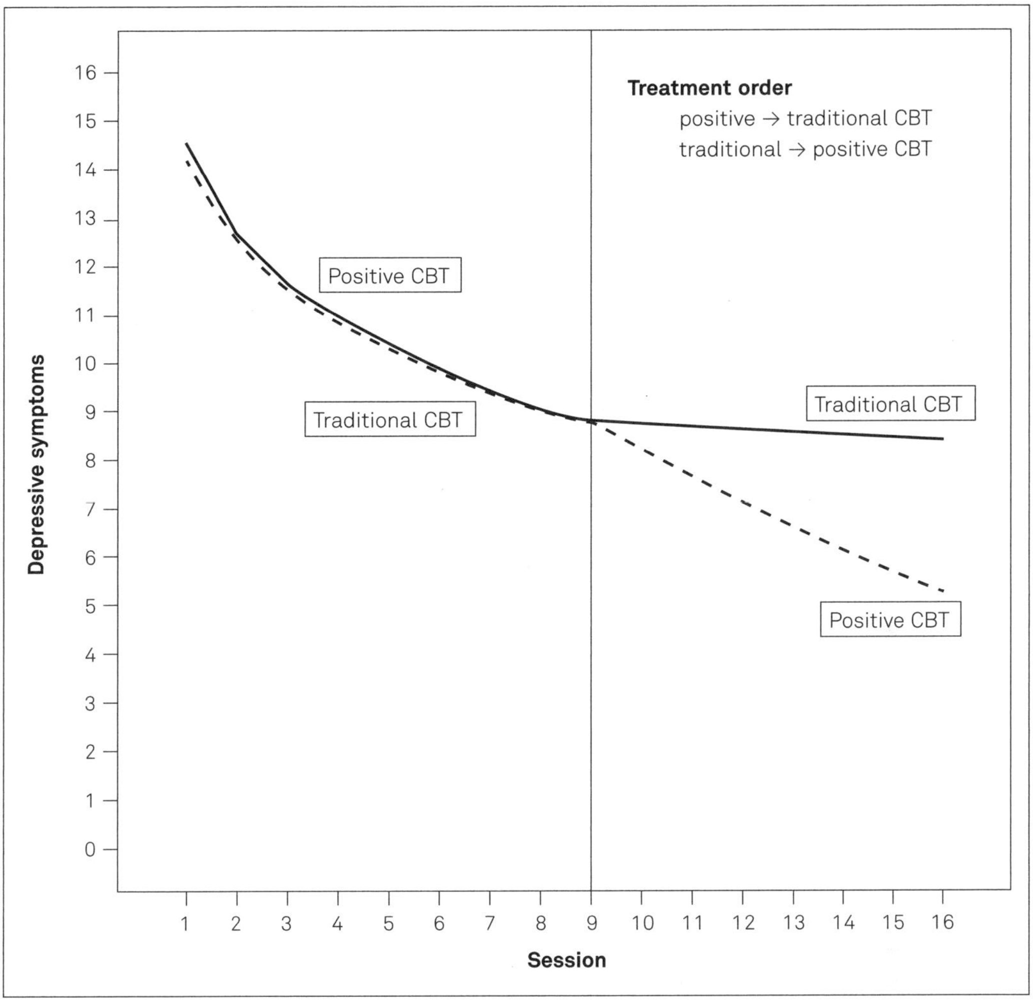

Figure 2 Comparison of the improvement of depressive symptoms during positive CBT and traditional CBT

For participants who started with positive CBT and then switched to traditional CBT, the improvement stagnated during traditional CBT. For participants who started with traditional CBT and then switched to positive CBT, the improvement of depressive complaints during the second phase continued, to a similar degree, as during the first phase (see Figure 2).

Additional analyses showed that significantly more *clinically significant* changes in depressive symptoms and negative affect occurred during positive CBT, compared with traditional CBT. "Clinically significant" means that this analysis only took into account major and relevant improvements – improvements that were not only statistically significant, but also clinically relevant. For example, depressive symptoms (scored on a scale of 0–27, with 0 representing no symptoms and 27 representing a lot of symptoms) had to be lowered by more than 7.8 points to be considered clinically significant. During positive CBT, 57% of clients experienced clinically significant improvement of depressive symptoms (averaged over the first and last phase, thus irrespective of the order of positive and traditional CBT), compared with only 24% during traditional CBT.

Significantly more clinically significant changes were also as measured with the Remission from Depression Questionnaire (Zimmerman et al., 2013), which captures not only decreases in depressive symptoms, but also increases in positive mental health, coping ability, functioning, life satisfaction, and sense of well-being. These clinically significant change effects were independent of the treatment phase: Positive CBT performed significantly better regarding clinically significant change on these measures than traditional CBT across both phases.

For positive affect and other indicators of positive mental health, we found no statistically significant differences between the two conditions. Given that these questionnaires were administered less often than those for the depressive symptoms (every fourth session only), this may have been caused by a lack of statistical power. Across all effect sizes (for positive affect, optimism, happiness, positive mental health, and remission from depression), the effects were on average 35% larger for positive CBT than for traditional CBT (although, as mentioned, the difference was not statistically significant).

We observed significantly less dropout among clients with positive CBT (three out of 24 dropped out) compared with clients who started with traditional CBT (nine out of 25). Most of the dropout in the group that started with traditional CBT took place during the first eight sessions (during traditional CBT). On the other hand, this group (with the order traditional CBT followed by positive CBT) had the best effects overall, which renders the interpretation of the results somewhat difficult.

Results of the Qualitative Study

The first 12 clients who participated in our study (six clients who started with traditional CBT, and six clients who started with positive CBT) were interviewed about their experience with both forms of CBT at the end of the therapy process (Geschwind et al., 2020). We asked what clients thought about traditional and positive CBT prior to therapy, and about their expectations and possible preconceptions. We also wanted to know whether they preferred positive or traditional CBT after completing both forms of therapy and, if there was a preference, what the reasons behind their preferences were.

The interviews showed that clients fell into three groups regarding their initial expectations and preconceptions of positive CBT: skeptical, mocking, and carefully positive. Clients who were skeptical thought that the purpose of therapy should be to talk about their problems instead of about positive things. Clients who were mocking were influenced by widely held beliefs ("Stand in front of the mirror and tell myself how well I'm doing everything").

Carefully positive clients, on the other hand, thought that a (more) positive focus might help them, given how negative they felt about their lives. Note that the clients who were initially skeptical or mocking changed their minds after their experience with positive CBT and were very enthusiastic about it afterwards.

Regarding their eventual preferences, nine out of 12 clients indicated that, given a choice between positive and traditional CBT, they would opt for positive CBT, sometimes supplemented with elements of traditional CBT. Nobody chose traditional CBT. The other three participants, somewhat surprisingly, experienced no difference between the two forms of treatment. Two of these three participants had difficulty freeing up time for the therapy; they went through the treatment passively and could not remember most of it. The third participant reported that she continued to apply the positive CBT exercises even after the transition to traditional CBT, a phenomenon called *carry-over effect*. All of the examples she mentioned of influential moments of therapy came from positive CBT.

The reasons given for a strong preference for positive CBT indicate a central role for positive emotions. Four themes emerged from the analysis. Positive CBT contributed to

1. feeling better and more empowered;
2. experiencing the upward spiral effect of positive emotions;
3. identifying baby steps; and
4. (re)discovering optimism.

We discuss all four themes below.

Feeling Better and More Empowered

Regarding the first theme, clients indicated that they experienced the focus on better moments, their strengths, and the work toward the self-formulated goal as pleasant – even in the context of acute depression. The fact that there were actually many more positive things in their lives than they had initially thought was a game changer: It contributed to an immediate positive mood change and gave them energy. In the quote below, a client describes an important moment in his therapy. Despite the unobtrusive content of the conversation and the fact that the client appears hesitant – probably because the therapist was the first to label his behavior as positive – he started to look at himself in a more positive light from that moment on.

Client:
And then the therapist said: "And what else? What else is better?" And I said, "Like what?"

Therapist: What do you think about the fact that you went grocery shopping? And cooking? You just said you cooked for yourself?

Client: Yes, I made spaghetti and it was tasty.

Therapist: So you cooked your own meal!

Client: Mwah, otherwise I wouldn't get anything to eat.

Therapist: You could have bought a ready-made meal?

Client: No, those are inedible.

Therapist: And so you started to cook yourself.

Client: Yes.

Therapist: To me, that is something positive. What do you think?

Client: Okay.

> Client:
> The biggest change is that I can now also talk positively about myself. People gave me compliments, but I couldn't do anything with them, the compliments didn't register with me. Now, I am working very hard on that. Now, when someone gives me a compliment, I notice: "Oh, that was a compliment," and I give a social answer. I also think of a compliment to say, such as: "You look nice today." I now get very different conversations; they are much more about the good things in life.

Many clients also described how empowering it was to think and talk in detail about their goal. They started looking more at what they wanted themselves instead of conforming to what others (boss, partner, family, friends) wanted from them. They linked this change to the fact that they first thought carefully about their goal, and subsequently made choices that brought them closer to their goal.

> Client:
> During every session, we talked about my goal and how far I had come: What rating do you give your current situation? This way you are more aware of your goal and become more active: What do I want, what went well today, what worked, what did not yet go well, and what can I do about it? I have discovered that it is important to talk about myself and about what I want, from a first-person perspective.

Experiencing the Upward Spiral Effect of Positive Emotions

According to the broaden-and-build theory of positive emotions (Fredrickson, 2003, 2009), positive emotions not only feel pleasant, but they also have valuable long-term effects. Positive emotions stimulate us to look at our environment in a more open way, to playfully explore and try new things, and to invest in social relationships, thereby leading to upward spiral effects (Garland et al., 2010). The *undoing hypothesis* related to the broaden-and-build theory additionally states that positive emotions undo negative emotions and other consequences of stress (Fredrickson et al., 2000).

In the interviews, many clients described how they noticed this undoing effect in their daily lives:

> Client:
> When you are in such a positive flow, problems feel less serious, they don't bother you so much. They feel much less stressful because you are more focused on positive things. That is why problems sort of shift to the background.

Clients also connected the therapy conversations about better moments and strengths to drastic changes inside and outside of therapy. One client described how positive CBT gave her a "protective suit of armor," enabling her to deal with problems and negative emotions in a better way. The biggest change was that – for the first time in her 60-year life – she became aware that she was actually a valuable person. She mentioned that others also perceived this change: She received many compliments about the fact that she now had a much more open and outgoing appearance, took initiative, and dared to take up space.

Identifying Baby Steps

Identifying *baby steps* – small steps forward – and appreciating and celebrating them, was unusual for many clients. In the past, they had regularly struggled with not achieving their goal and therefore felt they had been "failing" again. The same thing happened with clients who, outside therapy, tried, as they phrased it, "to think positively." Change should be easy, they thought, and when they did not succeed, they quit. The stories of these clients show that positivity requires endurance, but also yields a lot.

> Client:
> Perceiving small positive changes, or things that are already going well, and seeing that these are valuable ... that was something that I found extremely difficult to do. I really tried to look for these little things. In the beginning I just didn't see them. It actually took several sessions before it became easier.

By focusing attention, in a structured way, on what is better in their lives (even just a little bit) and positively reinforcing every little step, the therapist helps the client to continue practicing and to sustain improvements. Also for the CBT therapists in our research, for whom positive CBT was also a new approach, it was valuable to be reminded from time to time that positive CBT requires a different mindset, a different way of looking at things. Clients were initially also struggling with this other mindset. The therapist's ability to radiate confidence and set a good example can help clients to overcome this struggle. In our study, we did not investigate how the therapists themselves experienced positive CBT. It would be useful to evaluate therapists' experience in another qualitative study.

(Re)discovering Optimism

The (re)discovery of optimism was a recurring topic in the interviews. We explicitly write (re)discovery, because optimism was a revelation for some clients, while others described how they had been optimists prior to the depressive episode, but had lost their optimism during it. The question whether clients with an (originally) optimistic attitude would benefit more from positive CBT than clients who considered themselves lifelong pessimists came up during supervision of therapists participating in the study. Our impression was that everyone could take advantage of the (re)discovery of optimism; and that pessimistic clients may benefit even more from practicing an optimistic outlook on life. Nevertheless, discovering the potential of a more positive focus took longer for convinced pessimists, and in those cases demanded more perseverance from therapists. Note that this conclusion is based on our experience as therapists and supervisors – we did not investigate it formally.

> Client:
> I used to be a complete pessimist ... this was a shock therapy for me! In the end there were so many positive things that I never perceived before. Now I am completely convinced: I choose to embrace the radical perspective of looking things in a positive light.

> Client:
> Positive CBT appealed to me because I always had a positive outlook on life. [Laughing] You wouldn't say it in the context of a depression but I really am a positive person. That's why I thought this might help to become more positive again in my life.

> Client:
> As an example ... your slipper breaks. You may find that very annoying and let it ruin your entire day, but you can also say to yourself: "It was poor quality and at a certain point, they do break." That's it: convert everything into something positive. If something goes well, you might think: "I worked very hard for it." And not: "When will the bad stuff come."

Conclusions

In summary, our research showed that:

- A focus on the preferred future, the better moments (exceptions), personal strengths, and positive emotions reduces depressive complaints and negative emotions effectively.
- There was significantly less initial dropout with positive CBT followed by traditional CBT, than when the treatments were arranged the other way around. Due to the cross-over design (comparison of both forms of treatment within one treatment), this finding is difficult to interpret, because the group that started with traditional CBT achieved better results overall, but also had the highest dropout rate;
- Clients perceived positive CBT to be more pleasant than traditional CBT.

The results of this first research into positive CBT are promising. However, further research is needed. Further studies could compare treatment with either traditional CBT *or* positive CBT in a randomized controlled trial. Follow-up measurements (after 6 months, 1 year, and 2 years) could then investigate differences in behavior maintenance between positive and traditional CBT. Although positive CBT is essentially transdiagnostic, the effectiveness of positive CBT for diagnoses other than depressive disorder needs evaluation.

A qualitative study could investigate not only the experiences of clients, but also the experiences of therapists working with positive CBT. It would also be interesting to study the effectiveness of the group treatment protocol (see Chapter 4), and find the development of a treatment protocol especially designed for children and adolescents important.

Chapter 3
Individual Positive CBT Protocol

One doesn't discover new lands without consenting to lose sight of the shore for a very long time.

André Gide, French writer

Introduction

This chapter presents the individual positive CBT protocol. It can be seen as "discovering new lands" within the CBT field. And just as there is not one form of traditional CBT, there is not one form of positive CBT. By popular demand, we describe the protocol in eight sessions, as we developed and applied it in our research (see Chapter 2).

We have chosen exercises from the positive psychology movement that we think are best suited to the diagnosis of major depressive disorder (focus of our research group) and exercises that were already available 6 years ago, when we started our research. In the case of other diagnoses, or under other different circumstances, you might choose some other exercises, as we did in the treatment protocol for positive CBT in a group (see Chapter 4). However, for research purposes it is important to continue applying the same protocol, because otherwise the results cannot be compared. We developed the individual treatment protocol at Maastricht University, the Netherlands, and applied it in our study to 49 outpatients suffering from a major depressive disorder.

Clients rated positive CBT as very pleasant (see their quotes in this book). We described the results of our qualitative and quantitative research in Chapter 2.

> Client:
> I really enjoyed the positive sessions. I looked forward to them every week. She [the therapist] also stimulated my thinking, which was very nice. I think it is very difficult to change your thought pattern yourself. Especially in the beginning, I needed someone who invited me to see positive things in life. In the end, I managed to do this more and more by myself.

Client: It wasn't like: I have to go to the psychologist. It was like: Oh nice! We could really laugh together. It wasn't like: "What has been bothering you?" as you see on TV, lying on the couch and stuff like that. Yes, it felt very positive. I didn't have to feel ashamed; I really felt I could tell her everything and that she did not say [in an accusing voice]: Yes, you lack that, and that. She also talked about her sons, I thought that was very positive, because it is different from: I am your therapist and you don't have to know anything about me. It wasn't just a session, it was also very enjoyable. We certainly worked hard and it has been very helpful. And at one point, she said: "Look, you taught me something again!" I really liked that!

About Diagnostics

Positive CBT is transdiagnostic. By focusing on the preferred future or outcome (what does the client see as the best treatment result; what does the client want to see instead of the problem?) and on what works in the client's life, there is no need to distinguish between diagnoses.

As we implemented the treatment protocol with clients who suffered from a major depressive disorder, as mentioned earlier, there are exercises in this protocol which we found to be especially useful for clients suffering from low mood. As an example: we included the exercise "Optimistic Thinking Style" (Session 6), because people suffering from a major depressive disorder often have a pessimistic thinking style. This exercise can also be used with other disorders, or you may replace it with another exercise, as is done in the group protocol (see Chapter 4).

In this chapter we give a short explanation of the exercises and homework suggestions. As stated earlier (Section 1.3), we prefer the term "suggestions" instead of "tasks" or "assignments." We highlight the central homework suggestion: filling in the Diary of Better Moments (see Figure 3). This homework suggestion applies to all sessions (except Session 1).

Date	What happened?	What was better/ less bad?	What did I do differently?	What did I think/ feel differently?	What did I do to make that happen?

Figure 3 Diary of Better Moments.

In every subsequent session, the therapist asks about the client's observations of these better moments.

We then provide a brief overview of each session (see Table 1). Finally, we describe each session in great detail. You may use this protocol as a cookbook. As mentioned in the Preface, you will also find two "Clients' Workbooks" in the Appendices – one for individual and one for group positive CBT (Appendix 1 and Appendix 2). Therapists can download and print out the workbooks for their clinical work (please see the Appendix for more details).

Table 1 Brief overview of the treatment protocol for individual positive CBT

Session	Activities	Homework suggestions
Session 1	1 Welcome and building rapport, with a focus on client's strengths, values, and preferences 2 Explain the rationale of positive CBT 3 Ask about *pretreatment change* (what is better or different since client made the appointment?) 4 Ask the *miracle question* or other questions about the client's goal 5 Evaluate the collaborative relationship 6 Explain exercise "Your Best Possible Self" (King, 2001) 7 Explain exercise "Three Blessings" (Seligman et al., 2005) 8 Request client's feedback	1 Observe daily what goes well (enough) in your life. What does not need to change, or should not even change? 2 Exercise: "Your Best Possible Self" 3 Daily exercise: "Three Blessings"
Sessions 2–8	1 Start all sessions with opening question about progress, "What is better?" 2 Focus on exceptions, (small) successes and the client's contribution to make those exceptions happen, using EARS (De Jong & Berg, 2002) 3 Ask *scaling questions* to assess progress 4 Ask *competency questions*, "How did you do that?" and 'How do you cope?' 5 Discuss the homework suggestions, unless the client has not done any of them 6 Do the in-session exercises (see specific suggestions for each session). Do not do the proposed exercise when the client does not want to do it, or when you need more time to use EARS properly	

Table 1 continued

	7 Invite the client to start keeping the Diary of Better Moments (exceptions to the problem and/or the moments where there is already a glimpse of the preferred future) 8 Ask the client if they might find it useful to do a specific homework suggestion. If so, explain the suggestion and check if they have any questions 9 At the end of every session: request the client's feedback using the SRS (Duncan, 2010), including the question, "What can I (as your therapist) do better or different in the next session?" All exercises and homework suggestions will now be discussed per session	
	Suggestions for themes and exercises per session	**Homework suggestions**
Session 2	1 See to it that the goal formulation from Session 1 is stated in positive, concrete, and realistic terms (also use the results from exercise "Your Best Possible Self") 2 Ask scaling questions to find out where on a scale from 10 to 0 (10 being the ideal situation and 0 being the opposite) the client wants their situation to be in the preferred future, and then where on the scale the client would rate their current situation 3 Use further scaling questions to identify what progress the client has made and what next steps will look like 4 Consider asking scaling questions regarding the client's motivation, hope, and/or confidence that they will reach their goal 5 Explain exercise "Positive Self-Portrait"	1 Diary of Better Moments 2 Start making a Positive Self-Portrait
Session 3	1 Make topographic analyses of Better Moments, together with the client 2 Make positive FBAs of Better Moments, together with the client 3 Explain the VIA Character Strengths Survey	1 Diary of Better Moments 2 Fill in the VIA Character Strengths Survey online 3 Finish your Positive Self-Portrait

Table 1 continued

Session 4	1 Discuss the Positive Self-Portrait (homework started in Session 2) 2 Discuss the VIA Character Strengths Survey and how the client may use their top five to experience more well-being 3 Explain exercise "Create Powerful Beliefs"	1 Diary of Better Moments 2 Visualize daily your Powerful Beliefs
Session 5	1 Introduce "self-compassion" (Gilbert, 2010) 2 Do "Self-Compassion" exercise together 3 Explain exercise "Acts of Kindness" (Lyubomirsky, 2008)	1 Diary of Better Moments 2 Daily "Self-Compassion" exercise 3 Do 1 day each week: five acts of kindness
Session 6	1 Introduce "optimism" 2 Do exercise "Optimistic Thinking Style," together with the client (Seligman, 2002) 3 Do exercise "Upward Arrow Technique," together with the client	1 Diary of Better Moments 2 Daily exercise "Optimistic Thinking Style"
Session 7	1 Introduce "gratitude" 2 Discuss which three people the client is grateful for 3 Do exercise "Gratitude in Four Steps" 4 Explain Gratitude Letter	1 Diary of Better Moments 2 Do exercise "Gratitude in Four Steps" 3 Write Gratitude Letter and read the letter to that person
Session 8	1 Make plan for behavior maintenance 2 Request client's feedback for all eight sessions	1 Finish list of three times 50 things for behavior maintenance at home

Note. CBT = CBT = cognitive behavioral therapy; EARS = Elicit, Amplify, Reinforce, Start again; FBA = functional behavioral analyses; SRS = Session Rating Scale..

About the Exercises

The treatment protocol allows you to be flexible with regard to the exercises. They are suggestions, intended to invite clients to do the exercises. Clients may also, in consultation with the therapist, continue to do an exercise longer than initially planned and/or skip an exercise if they think it is not useful. The most important thing is that you, as their therapist, pay extensive attention to the better moments (exceptions) since the previous session and the clients' contribution to this, based on their Diary of Better Moments. There is no need to race through the program just to finish all of the exercises. If your clients require more time, let them have it. In cases where they think some parts are not really useful, allow them to skip those parts. We invite you, as their therapist, to read the Client's Workbook for individual positive CBT first, because it contains lots of information about the exercises, homework suggestions, and the actual wording you may use (Appendix 1).

About the Homework Suggestions

In the many supervision sessions that took place during the research period, the question was raised, what can you as a therapist do in case clients do not do the homework suggestions? This happens regularly. Explain to your client calmly that many clients have benefitted from the particular homework suggestion – and that therefore it also might help them. Invite clients to follow a certain suggestion, but always ask their opinion first. Do they want to do any homework at all? Are they motivated to do this particular suggestion? It is important that clients feel they have an opportunity to make choices. If clients do not want to do (extra) homework, then respect their choice. But let them know that every subsequent session you will invite them again to tell you about the better moments in their lives and their contribution to them, and to keep on monitoring these exceptions (see Chapter 1). Keeping a Diary of Better Moments is the most essential homework suggestion. Except for the first session, please repeat this suggestion in all eight sessions. If a client has not kept the diary, the therapist will still talk during the session about any exceptions the client remembers. The therapist asks questions about details of these exceptions to give them more weight – for example, "What exactly happened?" "How did you manage to do that?" and/or "How did you decide to do that?" (see Table 1 for a brief overview of all eight sessions).

Resistance

Within positive CBT, we assume that clients who have not done the homework suggestions always have a good reason for not doing it. It is their way of showing that this suggestion was not a good fit. In this way, there is always collaboration. If you see collaboration, you cannot see resistance; if you see resistance, you cannot see collaboration. Validate (instead of disqualify) their collaboration: "You must have a good reason for not having done the homework, please tell me more."

Even if they have not kept the diary, surely they have often noticed certain things or have been thinking about it. As therapist, you may ask about this and compliment them on all of their observations. If a client finds a homework suggestion difficult, validate and normalize this, and say, "Yes, it may be difficult, especially at the start of therapy – that's OK." Every attempt counts; it is about small baby steps forward, not about great leaps forward overnight.

Furthermore, the therapists who participated in the study sometimes found it difficult themselves to perform some of the exercises. During supervision, they were invited to first do the exercises themselves to observe the impact they might have – for example, some therapists found it difficult to ask a few important others to send them three written stories, in which those persons explained how the therapist contributed positively to their life (see exercise "Positive Self-Portrait," Sessions 2–4).

It is important to regularly repeat the rationale for the homework suggestions – for example, for the Diary of Better Moments. You might say, for example:

> I want to invite you to look at the better moments, because they contain the keys to find out what works for you, in your situation, at this point in time. Whether you write these moments down – or you may draw them – or just remember them, we will look for these keys together in therapy. And then it is just a matter of doing more of what works for you, in order to create a new and better life!

About the Diary of Better Moments

Invite clients from the end of the second session and all subsequent sessions (see Figure 3) to pay attention until the next session to those moments when things are (slightly) better or (slightly) less bad, on a daily basis. Also invite them to observe what they are doing differently at those moments, or what they are thinking and feeling differently, and what they did to make that happen. The Diary of Better Moments can also be found in the Client's Workbook (see Appendix 1).

> Client:
> My mother did the same. She checked every day what went well or what was better, even though she was very ill. It surprised me that my mother could stay so positive. Now that she is deceased, I think: She is my mother. Some part of my mother must be inside of me: I must be able to do that too.

> Client:
> I now search for small positive things every day and write them down, even though I think nothing special happened. I am surprised to find more and more positive thoughts. I recently enjoyed the sun on my face so much that I was shocked! Normally I really don't care, but now I thought: Ah, how nice! And I meant it too, it happened very spontaneously.

Overview of the Individual Positive CBT Protocol

Below you will find the individual positive CBT protocol. The protocol contains eight sessions (see Table 1). Each session lasts about 50 minutes. This is a brief overview; you will find the details later in this chapter. For more detailed information about all exercises and homework suggestions, we recommend Fredrike Bannink's previous book *Practicing Positive CBT,* on this subject (Bannink, 2012).

> Client:
> As an example.... it was raining today. In the past I would get annoyed, and stay annoyed: Oh no, it's raining, I'll be soaking wet. Now I think: Well, how can I solve this? I can't change anything about the rain, so I'll have to find a way to go out in a pleasant manner. Then, at least, I won't feel rotten anymore. This is a very simple example, but those are the things that I now deal with differently, every day. And I could name a hundred things that are different now.

Overview of the Sessions

In this section, we describe all of the explanations, exercises, and homework suggestions belonging to each session. As we mentioned earlier, we realize that you may consider our choice of exercises as somewhat arbitrary. In this protocol, we have aligned the exercises as much as possible for clients suffering from a major depressive disorder, because our research was aimed at this group of clients.

We have given specific attention to constructs such as self-compassion, altruism, optimism, and gratitude, but not to constructs such as hope (except for the opening question, "What are your best hopes?") and resilience. In the end, positive CBT is aimed at discovering and increasing hope and resilience, not only in the case of depression, but for all mental disorders. Furthermore, these constructs are often related. As an example, optimism, positive affect, and gratitude all contribute to resilience.

In Appendix 1 of this book you will find the Client's Workbook for Positive CBT With Individuals.

Please note that if an exercise introduced in a session is used again in a later session, then we have repeated the instructions, but highlighted these with a thin black vertical line.

> Client:
> These were really cheerful moments. That you believe, for the first time really start to believe, in yourself. The exercise of asking positive feedback from other people [Positive Self-Portrait] made me realize that how I begin to see myself now is not just in my head, no. It is being confirmed by others. I never realized that people see me the way they wrote in their letters . . . positive, cheerful, taking initiative, you name it ....all very positive things. That realization is growing slowly during therapy. When it is confirmed by the people you love, it is much more impressive and has a greater effect.

Session 1

1. Welcome and Building Rapport With a Positive Start

Warmly welcome the client and ask questions such as, "What do you do in your daily life?" (work, school, and private), "What are you good at?" and "What do you like about the things you do?" The aim of these questions is to make the introduction a positive one, to build a positive collaborative relationship (rapport), and to get a positive image with regard to the client (who is always much more than the problems they experience). Such a positive introduction also serves as an icebreaker and indicates that this therapy might be different from what they expect, based on previous treatments or their ideas about psychotherapy.

2. Give the Rationale for Positive CBT

Discuss the following with the client (you can read it verbatim, or say it in your own words): "We will work with positive cognitive behavioral therapy: positive CBT. We are not going to focus on what's wrong and what is not working. We will focus on your strengths and what works in your life instead – because these are the keys to start feeling better. We will also actively build on your well-being, positive thoughts and positive feelings. Positive thoughts and feelings are important to experience more well-being. They act as a buffer against the impact of setbacks, and motivate us to explore the environment, make contacts, and see and use opportunities. Research shows that people who suffer from depression experience fewer positive feelings. Moreover, it appears that for the recovery of depression the (re)creation of positive feelings, such as hope and gratitude, is more important than reducing negative feelings, such as fear and feeling sad. Research also shows that positive feelings protect us against relapse. Therefore, positive feelings are not only pleasant, but also important.

"We will also pay ample attention to what your preferred future looks like, to your personal strengths, and to the moments that are a little bit better or less bad. In addition, we will be watchful for those times when a glimpse of what you want to see (your preferred future), instead of the problem, is already visible. This is important, because these better moments (exceptions) are the keys to better functioning and more well-being – the keys to your new and better life.

"Positive CBT requires a different way of looking at things – you might say a different mindset. At the start it may feel a bit strange if you previously had psychotherapy that mainly looked at problems and how to repair them. In positive CBT you certainly do not have to pretend there are no problems or that you are not allowed to talk about them. However, we will focus first and foremost on what you want to see, instead of the problems, and at which moments this is already the case, even just a little bit, and how you succeed in making this happen."

3. Ask About Pretreatment Change

Research shows that prior to the first session two thirds of clients can already give a positive answer to the question about *pretreatment change* (Weiner-Davis et al., 1987). Ask your client, "Many clients notice that in the time between making the appointment and the first session, things begin to improve already or are a bit better. What did you notice that is different about your situation, during this time?" "What else did you notice?" and "What else?"

4. Ask Questions About Goal Formulation (in Positive, Concrete, and Realistic Terms)

Several questions are possible when asking about the goal of the client. You may ask, "What are your best hopes?" "What else are you hoping for?" and "What else?" The next question would be, "What difference will it make when all your best hopes are met?" and "What difference will make it for important others?" Or you may ask, "What will be the best result of this therapy?" or "What do you want to see instead of the problem?" Another way of inviting the client to describe their goal is to ask the *miracle question*, "Suppose a miracle happens while you are asleep tonight – the miracle being that tomorrow all problems are gone – but you didn't know because you were sleeping. What will be the first thing tomorrow morning that will tell you that this miracle has happened?" "What else will you notice?" and "What else?" (note: solution-focused questions are asked in the unconditional future tense, so we prefer "will," not "would.")

Also *scaling questions* are useful, where 10 means the ideal situation, and 0 means the opposite. The order of asking scaling questions is as follows. First, ask where on the scale the client wants their situation to be when they have reached their preferred future (or the end of therapy). Then, which mark on the scale does the client give their current situation, and how is it that it is not lower? Then, "What does a higher mark look like?" and "What will be different?" And finally, ask, "How can they get there?" or "What and/or who may be useful to get to a higher mark?"

5. Evaluate the Collaborative Relationship in Relation to the Goal

Do you have a visitor, complainant, or customer relationship with your client (see Chapter 1)? (Note: this is an estimate of the *alliance* between therapist and client; it is not a characteristic of the client. This evaluation is important because it offers a good indication of the client's motivation to change.)

- Clients with whom you have a *visitor relationship* come involuntary; they are mandated (there is a referrer who thinks it is necessary for them to come to you). Compliment them on their willingness to see you, and acknowledge the fact that they may be (somewhat) on the defensive side. Ask them what they think the referrer wants to see to be different at the end of therapy. Invite them to share their reactions with you and describe what they are willing to do. Do not give homework suggestions.
- Clients with whom you have a *complainant relationship* come voluntarily, but do not see themselves as part of the problem and/or the solution: Someone else or something else needs to change. Acknowledge their suffering, and ask a specific set of solution-focused questions to invite them to change themselves. Give only observational homework suggestions.

- Clients with whom you have a *customer relationship* also come voluntarily. They do see themselves as part of the problem and/or solution. They are motivated to change and may receive both observational and behavioral homework suggestions. Remember: As long as you are not part of the solution, you are part of the problem!

This classification largely determines the course of the sessions and the homework suggestions – for example, as a rule, clients with whom you have a complainant relationship need much more acknowledgment (a useful question being, "How do cope with everything that is going on in your life?"), and only observational homework suggestions are suitable.

Ask if clients (except clients with whom you have a visitor relationship) are willing to do some homework between sessions. If yes, first explain each suggestion – for example, ask, "Between now and the next session, pay attention to what in your life you want to keep the way it is and what does not need to (or should not) change." The therapist assumes that there are always (positive) things that clients like to keep the way they are. This is an observational suggestion and therefore is also suitable for clients with whom you have a complainant relationship. We call this suggestion the *first session formula task.*

6. Explain the Exercise "Your Best Possible Self"

Research shows that this is a useful exercise for setting achievable and attractive goals, and that it increases optimism and hope (Meevissen et al., 2011). Say or read the following to your client:

> Imagine a moment in the future when you are at your best. Visualize this best possible self, a version of yourself that you are pleased with and which fascinates and interests you. Imagine you have worked hard and succeeded in achieving your life goals. Think of dreams that you want to realize using your own talents and potential. The point is not to think of unrealistic fantasies, but rather of goals that are positive, attainable, and within reason. After you get a clear image, write down the details. Writing down your thoughts and dreams helps to organize vague ideas and fragmented thoughts, so you can focus on concrete and real possibilities. Please write everything down in your Workbook and bring it to the next session.

7. Explain the Exercise "Three Blessings"

Research shows that doing this exercise even only for 1 week increases well-being immediately and continuously (even 6 months later; Seligman, 2011). Many clients think that this is a pleasant exercise and keep on doing it for longer than a week, but you do not have to.

Say or read this to your client:

> Every day, write down three good things that happened each day for a week. Those three things can be small (e.g., I went to bed early tonight, as I had planned) or large (e.g., the guy I've liked for months asked me out). Also write down how you contributed to those good things and what they say about you.

8. Request the Client's Feedback, Using the Session Rating Scale

Every time when using the GSRS, the follow-up question is, "What can I (as your therapist) and/or the group do differently or better the next session to get a higher score than today?" (see the Appendix in *Practicing Positive CBT*, Bannink, 2012; *Posttraumatic Success*, Bannink, 2014; and https:\\www.scottdmiller.com). If clients give very high scores, you may ask instead, "What should I and/or the group continue to do in order to receive the same high score, at the end of the next session, as you gave me and/or the group in this session?"

Homework Suggestions – Session 1

1. First session, formulate task: "Between now and the next session please pay attention to what you want to keep in your life as it is. What does not have to – or should not even – change?"
2. Do the exercise "Your Best Possible Self."
3. Do the exercise "Three Blessings."

Session 2

1. Ask the Opening Question About Progress: "What Is Better?"

Only if the client cannot name anything that is better, you may ask, "What is different?" Use the Diary of Better Moments for this.

The implicit suggestion behind the question, "What is better?" is *that* something is better and that one only needs to look at *what* it is that is better. Experience shows that if the therapist always starts with this opening question, clients come to expect this question and will come up with an answer sooner than they would otherwise. When therapists ask very precisely about a past period, these exceptions can almost always be found. These are the times when the problem might reasonably have happened but somehow did not, or the problem was less, or they are moments when clients were able to cope better and/or moments when there was already something visible of what they want to see instead of the problem (their preferred future).

Note that the question, "What is better?" – in the present tense – is different from "How did you do in the past week?" "What went well?" or "What went better?" Initially, it may require some courage to be 100% predictable as a therapist, asking this opening question about progress (which may be different from how you have been working until now).

2. Use EARS: Elicit, Amplify, Reinforce, and Start Again

Invite the client to share positive information, then expand this information by asking questions about the details, and reinforce this positive information by being attentive and giving indirect compliments – for example, ask, "How were you able to do this?" or "How did you come up with that good idea?"

After highlighting the first example, ask again, "What else is better?" and continue asking "And what else?" Keep repeating the question, "What else?" to invite clients to look further than they might do initially. The most beautiful and important exceptions often come after the first and second answers.

Another often successful solution-focused intervention is this: First ask very pessimistic or depressed clients, "Please tell me about the worst moment since the last session." Listen respectfully and acknowledge the impact of the situation, but do not ask questions about details. Then continue, "So the other moments must have been at least a little bit better. Please tell me more about those."

3. Ask Scaling Questions About Progress

With scaling questions, therapists help clients to describe complex and intuitive observations of their past experiences and future possibilities. In this Session 2, use scaling questions to get a clear and concrete vision of their goal. Stick to a fixed order while searching for positive differences, starting with the question about the goal – the preferred future or preferred outcome.

First, use scaling questions from 10 to 0, where 10 means the ideal situation, and 0 means the opposite. You do not have to ask any specific questions about 10 and 0: 10 just means all of their best hopes are met. Ask, "If 10 is the ideal situation, and 0 is the opposite, which number do you want to reach on that scale?" Their goal should be stated in realistic, concrete, and positive terms. Ask, "How exactly will your life be different?" and "What will you be doing differently?" inviting the client to give you a detailed description. Most clients will say that they want to reach a 7 or 8 on the scale.

The second question to ask is, "Where on the scale do you want your situation to be when you have finished this therapy?" The difference is the time perspective; the preferred future may be in a few years' time, but therapy is often shorter and therefore the feasibility of the goal might be different. You may start with a more general question, "Where do you want to end up on the scale?" and then ask, "Where on the scale do you want your situation to be at the end of therapy?" Or you may ask, "When can we stop meeting like this?" or "When is it not necessary to come here anymore?" Invite clients to give a detailed description of their preferred future from early in the morning until late in the evening. What does their new and better life look like exactly? (Bannink, 2010, 2014, 2015a, 2015b).

The third question is, "What mark or number on the 10–0 scale do you give your current situation?"

Then, fourth, ask, "How is it that this number is not lower than it is?" "What is working?" "What else?" and "What else?" These questions focus on the exceptions and the client's competencies. Clients only need to do more of what works. This means that the solution does not have to come from you as their therapist!

The fifth set of questions is, "What does one point higher on the scale look like?" "How will you notice that your situation is one point higher?" "What will others notice that is different?" "How will they react (differently)?" "Who will be the least surprised?" "What will be next signs of progress?" or "Who will be the first to notice?"

Finally, the sixth question is, "Who or what may be useful to reach a higher number?"

Tip: Keep the triangle, *behavior–cognition–emotion,* in mind when inviting clients to describe their preferred future. Focus on positive differences compared with the present or the past, by always mentioning the term "different" or "differently":

Behavior: "What will you be doing differently?" (in the preferred future). Also use questions from other perspectives. "What will a friend see you doing differently, or family, or colleagues?" "How will they react differently?"

Cognitions: "How will you be thinking differently?" "How will you talk differently to yourself?"

Emotions: "How will you be feeling differently?"

Ask Competency Questions

Ask *competency questions* during every session. Competency questions are a form of indirect compliments. They invite clients to tell a success story about themselves. Examples of competency questions are "How did you succeed in doing that?" "How did you decide to do that?" "How did you manage that?" "How did you come up with that good idea?" "How do you cope?" and "How do you keep your head above water?"

4. Discuss the Homework Suggestions

Ask clients what they think of the questions, "What do you want to keep in your life? What does not have to change – or what should not even change?" (first session formula task). Also discuss the exercise "Your Best Possible Self." Say to them, "Have you given this some further thought? What aspects of this exercise can we add to the earlier description of your goal, your preferred future?"

5. Discuss the Exercise "Three Blessings"

Research shows that doing this exercise even only for 1 week increases well-being immediately and continuously (even 6 months later; Seligman, 2011). Many clients think that this is a pleasant exercise and keep on doing it for longer than a week, but you do not have to.

Say or read this to your client, "Every day, write down three good things that happened each day for a week. Those three things can be small (e.g., I went to bed early tonight, as I had planned) or large (e.g., the guy I've liked for months asked me out). Also write down how you contributed to those good things and what they say about you."

6. Ask if the Client Wants to Do Some Homework Between This and the Next Session

If yes, then explain the homework suggestions (Homework Suggestions – Session 2).

7. Request the Client's Feedback, Using the SRS, and Ask the Follow-up Question

Use the SRS, and then ask the follow-up question, What can I as a therapist do differently or better next time? (see Session 1).

Homework Suggestions – Session 2

1. Invite the client to keep the Diary of Better Moments throughout the therapy: Say to them, "Every day until we see each other again, please pay attention to those moments in which things are a little bit better – or a little less bad – and write down in your Workbook what is different about those moments and what you are doing differently."
2. Ask the client to start making a Positive Self-Portrait: The client is invited to bring the Positive Self-Portrait to the fourth session, so they will have sufficient time to request positive feedback from other people.

Say:

> Ask at least five people who know you well to give you three written stories of instances when you did something positive in their life. If it is difficult to get written stories, it is also OK to receive them orally and write them down in your Workbook. But often a written story is the best.

Collect all stories and read them to identify common themes, surprises and insights. Summarize the stories as your Positive Self-portrait and come up with a plan: how can you use your specific talents and strengths optimally? Then inform important people in your life about your plans.

If you shy away from asking five (or more) people, it helps to reflect on the effect these conversations might have. You will get meaningful conversations with five (or more) people who are important to you; you will get positive reactions; you will probably get a valuable exchange about many domains of your personal and social life, work, spirituality, and so on. Think how valuable this may be for yourself, for important others and for your relationship with them.

Please bring your Positive Self-portrait to the fourth session, however, take your time; this self-portrait does not have to be totally complete by the next session.

Session 3

1. Ask the Opening Question About Progress: "What Is Better?"

Use the Diary of Better Moments.

2. Use EARS: Elicit, Amplify, Reinforce, Start Again

Invite the client to share positive information, then expand this information by asking questions about the details, and reinforce this positive information by being attentive and giving indirect compliments – for example, ask, "How were you able to do this?" or "How did you come up with that good idea?"

After highlighting the first example, ask again, "What else is better?" and continue asking "And what else?" Keep repeating the question, "What else?" to invite clients to look further than they might do initially. The most beautiful and important exceptions are often somewhat harder to find than the first and second answer.

Another often successful solution-focused question is this: First ask very pessimistic or depressed clients, "Please tell me about the worst moment since the last session." Listen respectfully and acknowledge the impact of the situation, but do not ask questions about details. Then continue, "So the other moments must have been at least a little bit better. Please tell me more about those."

3. Ask Scaling Questions About Progress

"What number on the 10 to 0 scale do you give your current situation?"

4. Discuss the Homework Suggestions

Find functional – helpful – cognitions and functional behavior.

5. Together With the Client, Make Topographical Analyses and Functional Behavioral Analyses

Topographic analyses (TAs) are concrete examples of better moments arising from the self-monitoring of exceptions. They serve as an aid for making positive *functional behavioral analyses* (FBAs).

Positive FBAs of desired behavior or of better moments can be formulated in an ABC scheme, which refers to *antecedents* (situation), *behaviors and beliefs* (associated with desired or less undesired behavior), and *consequences* of the desired or less undesired behavior (positive and – if present – also negative effects). See Chapter 5 (The Case of Carin) for an example of a positive FBA. Note that a negative C (consequence) is not obvious, but cannot be excluded either – for example, it may be that clients get less attention from the people around them once things are getting better.

6. Ask If the Client Wants to Do Some Homework Between This and the Next Session

If yes, then explain the homework suggestions (Homework Suggestions – Session 3).

7. Request Feedback From the Client

Request the client's feedback, using the SRS, and then ask the follow-up question.

Homework Suggestions – Session 3

1. Ask the client to continue the Diary of Better Moments.
2. Complete the VIA Character Strengths Survey: Invite the client to fill in the VIA Character Strengths Survey online (http://www.viacharacter.org/; see Chapter 1). Explain that "everyone has certain personal strengths. By completing the questionnaire, you can discover your strengths, so you may use them optimally. Through this link, you have to create an account first. Click on 'Register,' and then on 'Continue' on the next screen. You can save the records and send them to me, or print them yourself and bring them to the next session. It takes about 30 minutes to complete the Survey; however, it is certainly worth it."
   Motivate the client as follows, "It is very nice to see your personal strengths; it often gives a new perspective on yourself. Moreover, it is important to know what your top five character strengths are and to use those optimally to experience more well-being."
3. Ask the client to complete the Positive Self-portrait: Say to them, "Finish the Positive Self-portrait that you started earlier and bring it to the next session, even if it is not completely finished yet."

Session 4

1. Ask the Opening Question About Progress "What's Better?"

Use the Diary of Better Moments.

2. Use EARS: Elicit, Amplify, Reinforce, Start Again

Invite the client to share positive information, then expand this information by asking questions about the details, and reinforce this positive information by being attentive and giving indirect compliments – for example, ask, "How were you able to do this?" or "How did you come up with that good idea?"

After highlighting the first example, ask again, "What else is better?" and continue asking "And what else?" Keep repeating the question, "What else?" to invite clients to look further than they might do initially. The most beautiful and important exceptions are often somewhat harder to find than the first and second answer.

Another often successful solution-focused question is this: First ask very pessimistic or depressed clients, "Please tell me about the worst moment since the last session." Listen respectfully and acknowledge the impact of the situation, but do not ask questions about details. Then continue, "So the other moments must have been at least a little bit better. Please tell me more about those."

3. Ask Scaling Questions About Progress

With scaling questions, therapists help clients to describe complex and intuitive observations of their past experiences and future possibilities. In this Session 4, use scaling questions to get a clear and concrete vision of their goal. Stick to a fixed order while searching for positive differences, starting with the question about the goal – the preferred future or preferred outcome.

First, use scaling questions from 10 to 0, where 10 means the ideal situation, and 0 means the opposite. You do not have to ask any specific questions about 10 and 0: 10 just means all of their best hopes are met. Ask, "If 10 is the ideal situation, and 0 is the opposite, which number do you want to reach on that scale?" Their goal should be stated in realistic, concrete, and positive terms. Ask, "How exactly will your life be different?" and "What will you be doing differently?" inviting the client to give you a detailed description. Most clients will say that they want to reach a 7 or 8 on the scale.

The second question to ask is, "Where on the scale do you want your situation to be when you have finished this therapy?" The difference is the time perspective; the preferred future may be in a few years' time, but therapy is often shorter and therefore the feasibility of the goal might be different. You may start with a more general question, "Where do you want to end up on the scale?" and then ask, "Where on the scale do you want your situation to be at the end of therapy?" Or you may ask, "When can we stop meeting like this?" or "When is it not necessary to come here anymore?" Invite clients to give a detailed description of their preferred future from early in the morning until late

in the evening. What does their new and better life look like exactly? (Bannink, 2010, 2014, 2015a, 2015b).

The third question is, "What mark or number on the 10–0 scale do you give your current situation?"

Then, fourth, ask, "How is it that this number is not lower than it is?" "What is working?" "What else?" and "What else?" These questions focus on the exceptions and the client's competencies. Clients only need to do more of what works. This means that the solution does not have to come from you as their therapist!

The fifth set of questions is, "What does one point higher on the scale look like?" "How will you notice that your situation is one point higher?" "What will others notice that is different?" "How will they react (differently)?" "Who will be the least surprised?" "What will be next signs of progress?" or "Who will be the first to notice?"

Finally, the sixth question is, "Who or what may be useful to reach a higher number?"

Tip: Keep the triangle, *behavior–cognition–emotion,* in mind when inviting clients to describe their preferred future. Focus on positive differences compared with the present or the past, by always mentioning the term "different" or "differently":

Behavior: "What will you be doing differently?" (in the preferred future). Also use questions from other perspectives. "What will a friend see you doing differently, or family, or colleagues?" "How will they react differently?"

Cognitions: "How will you be thinking differently?" "How will you talk differently to yourself?"

Emotions: "How will you be feeling differently?"

4. Discuss the Homework Suggestions

Discuss the client's strengths based on the Positive Self-Portrait and the completed VIA Survey (pay particular attention to their top five). Explain that "all 24 strengths are shown on the survey. The order is important. The strengths at the top are the most fitting for you, the last ones the least. Therefore, we will not dwell on the lowest strengths for too long, but focus on the top five character strengths instead."

As an alternative (if clients have not completed the VIA Survey or have forgotten to bring it with them), compile a top five of their strengths with them as they see it, based on the 24 character strengths of Seligman and colleagues (see Table 2). Invite clients to choose three to five strengths and ask for some examples of how they have applied these strengths lately. If useful, also ask questions from the third-person perspective (family, close friends, colleagues). If clients cannot name anything or say little, inquire, "Suppose we were to ask some of your best friends what they think your five strengths are, what do you think they would say?"

Table 2 Classification of the six virtues and 24 character strengths (Peterson, 2006). Reproduced with permission of the Licensor through PLSclear

1. *Wisdom and knowledge:* Cognitive strengths that entail the acquisition and use of knowledge.
- *Creativity* (originality, ingenuity): Thinking of novel and productive ways to conceptualize and do things; includes artistic achievement but is not limited to it
- *Curiosity* (interest, novelty seeking, openness to experience): Taking an interest in ongoing experience for its own sake; finding subjects and topics fascinating; exploring and discovering
- *Judgment* (critical thinking): Thinking things through and examining them from all sides; not jumping to conclusions; being able to change one's mind in light of evidence; weighing all evidence fairly
- *Love of learning:* Mastering new skills, topics, and bodies of knowledge, whether on one's own or formally; obviously related to the strength of curiosity but goes beyond it to describe the tendency to add systematically to what one knows
- *Perspective* (wisdom): Being able to provide wise counsel to others; having ways of looking at the world that make sense to oneself and to other people

2. *Courage:* Emotional strengths that involve the exercise of will to accomplish goals in the face of opposition, external or internal
- *Bravery* (valor): Not shrinking from threat, challenge, difficulty, or pain; speaking up for what is right even if there is opposition; acting on convictions even if unpopular; includes physical bravery but is not limited to it
- *Perseverance* (persistence, industriousness): Finishing what one starts; persisting in a course of action in spite of obstacles; getting it out the door; taking pleasure in completing tasks
- *Honesty* (authenticity, integrity): Speaking the truth but more broadly presenting oneself in a genuine way and acting in a sincere way; being without pretense; taking responsibility for one's feelings and actions
- *Zest* (vitality, enthusiasm, vigor, energy): Approaching life with excitement and energy; not doing things halfway or halfheartedly; living life as an adventure; feeling alive and activated

3. *Humanity:* Interpersonal strengths that involve tending and befriending others
- *Love:* Valuing close relations with others, in particular those in which sharing and caring are reciprocated; being close to people
- *Kindness* (generosity, nurturance, care, compassion, altruistic love, niceness): Doing favors and good deeds for others; helping them; taking care of them
- *Social intelligence* (emotional intelligence, personal intelligence): Being aware of the motives and feelings of other people and oneself; knowing what to do to fit into different social situations; knowing what makes other people tick

4. *Justice*: Civic strengths that underlie healthy community life
- *Teamwork* (citizenship, social responsibility, loyalty): Working well as a member of a group or team; being loyal to the group; doing one's share
- *Fairness:* Treating all people the same according to notions of fairness and justice; not letting personal feelings bias decisions about others; giving everyone a fair chance.
- *Leadership:* Encouraging a group of which one is a member to get things done, and at the same time maintaining good relations within the group; organizing group activities and seeing that they happen.

Table 2 continued

5. *Temperance*: Strengths that protect against excess
- *Forgiveness:* Forgiving those who have done wrong; accepting the shortcomings of others; giving people a second chance; not being vengeful
- *Humility:* Letting one's accomplishments speak for themselves; not regarding oneself as more special than one is
- *Prudence:* Being careful about one's choices; not taking undue risks; not saying or doing things that might later be regretted
- *Self-regulation* (self-control): Regulating what one feels and does; being disciplined; controlling one's appetites and emotions

6. *Transcendence*: Strengths that forge connections to the larger universe and provide meaning
- *Appreciation of beauty and excellence* (awe, wonder, elevation): Noticing and appreciating beauty, excellence, and/or skilled performance in various domains of life, from nature to art to mathematics to science to everyday experience
- *Gratitude:* Being aware of, and thankful for, the good things that happen; taking time to express thanks
- *Hope* (optimism, future-mindedness, future orientation): Expecting the best in the future and working to achieve it; believing that a good future is something that can be brought about
- *Humor* (playfulness): Liking to laugh and tease; bringing smiles to other people; seeing the light side; making (not necessarily telling) jokes
- *Spirituality* (faith, purpose): Having coherent beliefs about the higher purpose and meaning of the universe; knowing where one fits within the larger scheme; having beliefs about the meaning of life that shape conduct and provide comfort

5. Discuss How Clients May Experience More Flow

Flow refers to the mental state in which we are completely absorbed by our pursuits and lose awareness of time (Csikszentmihalyi, 1990). Flow is associated with the pursuit of a certain purpose, such as making a painting or playing a musical instrument. This is realized if there is an optimal balance between the difficulty of the task and the specific competencies the person has. Furthermore, during flow, people can exceed their own level, learn faster, and gain new insights. Clients may experience more flow by using their top five signature strengths in a new area of life or by deploying those strengths more often in an already existing area (e.g., work or hobby).

6. Do the Exercise "Create Powerful Beliefs"

Explain that the following exercise is about creating powerful beliefs:
1. Think of something positive that you would like to think about yourself, but are not sure is correct (yet). Formulate your desired belief in a positive form. Make sure that it really suits you and that it is something you can actually do – for example, I am a confident person.

2. Ask yourself: What would someone who has this belief naturally do? Imagine a number of behaviors this person would show, and list them – for example, that person stands or sits upright, makes eye contact with other people, speaks clearly and loud enough, greets people upon arrival, gives their opinion, stands up for their opinion, is kind to others, is kind to themselves, smiles, does not necessarily do what others want them to do, but focuses on their own wishes and beliefs, wears clothes that they likes, breathes calmly, thinks that making mistakes can happen (and those do not say much about them), and when successful acknowledges that they have worked hard, taken initiatives, and so on.
3. Choose a situation in the future in which you want to have the desired belief – for example, when my parents-in-law are visiting us.
4. Choose behaviors from the list that show your desired belief and which fit into that particular situation – for example, I will wear clothes that I like and feel comfortable in, stand tall when opening the door, make eye contact with my mother-in-law, greet her in a friendly way, kiss her, shake my father-in-law's hand and say, "Come on in, nice to see you," speak clearly and loud enough, stand up for my own opinion, start a conversation myself, focus on myself, breath calmly (from my belly), and so on.
5. Imagine yourself in that situation while you behave that way. Look at the situation, like a movie scene, in which "your future you" behaves in accordance with your desired belief. If useful, change the scene till it is positive and really fits. (Tip: You may draw "film shots" with the client on a whiteboard or in their Workbook.)
6. Then return to the beginning of the scene. Step into the scene, and experience it as if it is really happening. Look at everything and everyone around you, and notice how you feel. Hear how you express your beliefs with certainty. Go through the whole scene.

Note that Step 6 is also the homework suggestion – to visualize this scene a couple of times on a daily basis. The more often the client practices, the easier the visualization becomes. Athletes also do this: Think of athletes who go over a bobsleigh track a thousand times in their heads, including making the corresponding movements. You may also ask clients to write down a couple of keywords on the whiteboard or in their Workbook. Repeat Steps 5 and 6 a few times.

7. Ask If the Client Wants to Do Some Homework Between This and the Next Session

If yes, then explain the homework suggestions (Homework Suggestions – Session 4).

8. Request the Client's Feedback, Using the SRS, and Ask the Follow-up Question

Use the SRS, and then ask the follow-up question: What can I as a therapist do differently or better next time?

Homework Suggestions – Session 4

1. Ask the client to continue the Diary of Better Moments.
2. Ask the client to Create Powerful Beliefs (see Step 6 in the exercise "Create Powerful Beliefs"): Ask the client to visualize the desired behavior in the desired situation a couple of times on a daily basis, using the exercise "Create Powerful Beliefs" (see Session 4.6).

Session 5

1. Ask the Opening Question About Progress "What's Better?"

Use the Diary of Better Moments.

2. Use EARS: Elicit, Amplify, Reinforce, Start Again

Invite the client to share positive information, then expand this information by asking questions about the details, and reinforce this positive information by being attentive and giving indirect compliments – for example, ask, "How were you able to do this?" or "How did you come up with that good idea?"

After highlighting the first example, ask again, "What else is better?" and continue asking "And what else?" Keep repeating the question, "What else?" to invite clients to look further than they might do initially. The most beautiful and important exceptions are often somewhat harder to find than the first and second answer.

Another often successful solution-focused question is this: First ask very pessimistic or depressed clients, "Please tell me about the worst moment since the last session." Listen respectfully and acknowledge the impact of the situation, but do not ask questions about details. Then continue, "So the other moments must have been at least a little bit better. Please tell me more about those."

3. Ask Scaling Questions About Progress

With scaling questions, therapists help clients to describe complex and intuitive observations of their past experiences and future possibilities. In this Session 5, use scaling questions to get a clear and concrete vision of their goal. Stick to a fixed order while searching for positive differences, starting with the question about the goal – the preferred future or preferred outcome.

First, use scaling questions from 10 to 0, where 10 means the ideal situation, and 0 means the opposite. You do not have to ask any specific questions about 10 and 0: 10 just means all of their best hopes are met. Ask, "If 10 is the ideal situation, and 0 is the opposite, which number do you want to reach on that scale?" Their goal should be stated in realistic, concrete, and positive terms. Ask, "How exactly will your life be different?" and "What will you be doing differently?" inviting the client to give you a detailed description. Most clients will say that they want to reach a 7 or 8 on the scale.

The second question to ask is, "Where on the scale do you want your situation to be when you have finished this therapy?" The difference is the time perspective; the preferred future may be in a few years' time, but therapy is often shorter and therefore the feasibility of the goal might be different. You may start with a more general question, "Where do you want to end up on the scale?" and then ask, "Where on the scale do you want your situation to be at the end of therapy?" Or you may ask, "When can we stop meeting like this?" or "When is it not necessary to come here anymore?" Invite clients to give a detailed description of their preferred future from early in the morning until late

in the evening. What does their new and better life look like exactly? (Bannink, 2010, 2014, 2015a, 2015b).

The third question is, "What mark or number on the 10–0 scale do you give your current situation?"

Then, fourth, ask, "How is it that this number is not lower than it is?" "What is working?" "What else?" and "What else?" These questions focus on the exceptions and the client's competencies. Clients only need to do more of what works. This means that the solution does not have to come from you as their therapist!

The fifth set of questions is, "What does one point higher on the scale look like?" "How will you notice that your situation is one point higher?" "What will others notice that is different?" "How will they react (differently)?" "Who will be the least surprised?" "What will be next signs of progress?" or "Who will be the first to notice?"

Finally, the sixth question is, "Who or what may be useful to reach a higher number?"

Tip: Keep the triangle, *behavior–cognition–emotion,* in mind when inviting clients to describe their preferred future. Focus on positive differences compared with the present or the past, by always mentioning the term "different" or "differently":

Behavior: "What will you be doing differently?" (in the preferred future). Also use questions from other perspectives. "What will a friend see you doing differently, or family, or colleagues?" "How will they react differently?"

Cognitions: "How will you be thinking differently?" "How will you talk differently to yourself?"

Emotions: "How will you be feeling differently?"

4. Discuss the Homework Suggestions

Discuss the exercise "Creating Powerful Beliefs."

5. Self-Compassion

Introduce the concept of *self-compassion.* You do not necessarily have to use the term "self-compassion." Some clients may find that term too difficult or woolly. You could also say, "Be kind to yourself, even when you are struggling." Compassion is the ability to feel involved with pain and suffering, both our own suffering and that of others. Feeling compassion for others is usually easy, but feeling self-compassion is often much harder. Ask for exceptions, "When in your life did you succeed in having (a little) self-compassion?"

6. Do the "Self-Compassion" Exercise Together

Say to the client, "This is an exercise to be more kind to yourself. Think back to a recent moment when you were sad. Have you found one? Then please go back to that moment for a while. Experience the sadness again. Sit quietly, close your eyes, engage in your breathing, and then imagine yourself as a compassionate person. When you can feel that expanding and growing inside you, then imagine you can see your own sad self in front of you. Look at their facial expression; note the feelings rushing through them. Just sit and feel compassion, and send compassionate feelings out to that sad self. Try to surround that sad self with compassion and understanding of the torment of sadness. For now, you are not trying to do anything other than experience compassion and acceptance for your grief. Imagine giving as much compassion and understanding as that sad part needs. You may want to imagine what happens to that sad part when it actually has all of the understanding and support it needs" (Gilbert, 2010, p. 171; in his exercise, Gilbert uses anxiety instead of sadness).

You may do the exercise twice, so clients are really able to feel it. You may also add a soothing movement: Ask clients to choose one themselves or ask them to put their hand on their shoulder. This is called cue conditioning and often has a positive effect. It is also possible to calm clients with words – for example, using a reassuring word or mantra, like "rest" or "relax."

7. Ask If the Client Wants to Do Some Homework Between This and the Next Session

If yes, then explain the homework suggestions (Homework Suggestions – Session 5).

8. Request the Client's Feedback, Using the SRS, and Ask the Follow-up Question

Use the SRS, and then ask the follow-up question: What can I as a therapist do differently or better next time?

Homework Suggestions – Session 5

1. Ask the client to continue the Diary of Better Moments.
2. Ask the client to do the "Self-Compassion" exercise daily (Step 6. Do the "Self-Compassion" Exercise Together).
3. Do the exercise "Five Acts of Kindness" (altruism): Introduce the exercise as follows: "Research shows that of all of the exercises which have been researched so far in the context of positive psychology, doing *acts of kindness* provides the most well-being. Do five acts of kindness all in one day (not one act a day, because then it may become boring and less effective). Do something that really makes a difference and requires some effort on your part, such as donating blood or helping your neighbors with their gardening, even if you do not really feel like it. Be creative and think about what people around you need the most. You may also turn the day, on which you do the five acts of kindness, into a ritual and create a fixed day every week in which you do this. Always find new acts of kindness that make a positive difference in the lives of others. Take some time to notice what difference this makes for others – and for yourself. Please write down all of your acts of kindness in your Workbook."

Session 6

1. Ask the Opening Question About Progress "What's Better?"

Use the Diary of Better Moments.

2. Use EARS: Elicit, Amplify, Reinforce, Start Again

Invite the client to share positive information, then expand this information by asking questions about the details, and reinforce this positive information by being attentive and giving indirect compliments – for example, ask, "How were you able to do this?" or "How did you come up with that good idea?"

After highlighting the first example, ask again, "What else is better?" and continue asking "And what else?" Keep repeating the question, "What else?" to invite clients to look further than they might do initially. The most beautiful and important exceptions are often somewhat harder to find than the first and second answer.

Another often successful solution-focused question is this: First ask very pessimistic or depressed clients, "Please tell me about the worst moment since the last session." Listen respectfully and acknowledge the impact of the situation, but do not ask questions about details. Then continue, "So the other moments must have been at least a little bit better. Please tell me more about those."

3. Ask Scaling Questions About Progress

With scaling questions, therapists help clients to describe complex and intuitive observations of their past experiences and future possibilities. In this Session 6, use scaling questions to get a clear and concrete vision of their goal. Stick to a fixed order while searching for positive differences, starting with the question about the goal – the preferred future or preferred outcome.

First, use scaling questions from 10 to 0, where 10 means the ideal situation, and 0 means the opposite. You do not have to ask any specific questions about 10 and 0: 10 just means all of their best hopes are met. Ask, "If 10 is the ideal situation, and 0 is the opposite, which number do you want to reach on that scale?" Their goal should be stated in realistic, concrete, and positive terms. Ask, "How exactly will your life be different?" and "What will you be doing differently?" inviting the client to give you a detailed description. Most clients will say that they want to reach a 7 or 8 on the scale.

The second question to ask is, "Where on the scale do you want your situation to be when you have finished this therapy?" The difference is the time perspective; the preferred future may be in a few years' time, but therapy is often shorter and therefore the feasibility of the goal might be different. You may start with a more general question, "Where do you want to end up on the scale?" and then ask, "Where on the scale do you want your situation to be at the end of therapy?" Or you may ask, "When can we stop meeting like this?" or "When is it not necessary to come here anymore?" Invite clients to give a detailed description of their preferred future from early in the morning until late in the evening. What does their new and better life look like exactly? (Bannink, 2010, 2014, 2015a, 2015b).

The third question is, "What mark or number on the 10–0 scale do you give your current situation?"

Then, fourth, ask, "How is it that this number is not lower than it is?" "What is working?" "What else?" and "What else?" These questions focus on the exceptions and the client's competencies. Clients only need to do more of what works. This means that the solution does not have to come from you as their therapist!

The fifth set of questions is, "What does one point higher on the scale look like?" "How will you notice that your situation is one point higher?" "What will others notice that is different?" "How will they react (differently)?" "Who will be the least surprised?" "What will be next signs of progress?" or "Who will be the first to notice?"

Finally, the sixth question is, "Who or what may be useful to reach a higher number?"

Tip: Keep the triangle, *behavior–cognition–emotion,* in mind when inviting clients to describe their preferred future. Focus on positive differences compared with the present or the past, by always mentioning the term "different" or "differently":

Behavior: "What will you be doing differently?" (in the preferred future). Also use questions from other perspectives. "What will a friend see you doing differently, or family, or colleagues?" "How will they react differently?"

Cognitions: "How will you be thinking differently?" "How will you talk differently to yourself?"

Emotions: "How will you be feeling differently?"

4. Discuss the Homework Suggestions

Discuss the exercises "Self-Compassion" and "Acts of Kindness."

5. Introduce the Concept of Optimism

Explain the difference between pessimistic and optimistic thinking styles and their consequences.

Say or read,

> Pessimistic people attribute negative events, in particular, to stable, global, and internal factors. They say, "Everything is going down the drain" (stable), "I will never be happy again" (global), and "I am good for nothing" (internal). They attribute positive events to temporary, specific, and external factors. They say, "That was only luck, it had nothing to do with me," when something positive happens.

> Optimistic people tend to think the opposite way. They attribute positive events to stable, global, and internal factors. When something positive happens, they believe that it does say something about to temporary, specific, and external factors – for example, "Meeting this deadline was unrealistic, given that I was ill with the flu." Thinking in a pessimistic way, especially about negative events, leads to hopelessness. The good news is that you can learn to be more optimistic and benefit from a more optimistic way of thinking.

Then do the exercise "Optimistic Thinking Style" together with the client. Say to them, "Optimism can be learned. This is an exercise to become more optimistic":

- Every evening, write a sentence in your Workbook about the best event of that day, as if it were caused by something stable, global, and internal (because I am ... or because I can ...) – for example, "Today a colleague offered to help me. This happened because I am someone who also helps others when needed."
- Every evening, also write a sentence about the worst event of the day, as if it were caused by something temporary, specific, and outside yourself (because X then Y) – for example, "Today I arrived late for my dentist appointment. This happened because the bus had an unexpectedly large delay. This is the only time I have been late."

6. Do the Exercise "Upward Arrow Technique" Together

Explain to the client:

> Think of something in your life you would like to see changed for the better. Then ask yourself, "Suppose something in that situation has improved, what difference will that make?" "What else will be different?" "What else?" "What will I be doing differently?" and "What else?" Discover that you can probably come up with more things than you first thought.

Other questions you may ask are, "Suppose it's possible for the situation to change, what will be different or better?" "What else?" "For yourself?" and "For others?" Or you may ask what the *best-case scenario* will be, "What is the best that could happen?" "Suppose that happens, what difference will that make?" and "In its turn, what difference will that make?"

The purpose of this exercise is to find out how many positive consequences one small change may generate. This exercise is often motivating and offers hope.

7. Ask If the Client Wants to Do Some Homework Between This and the Next Session

If yes, then explain the homework suggestions (Homework Suggestions – Session 6).

8. Request the Client's Feedback, Using the SRS, and Ask the Follow-up Question

Use the SRS, and then ask the follow-up question: What can I as a therapist do differently or better next time?

Homework Suggestions – Session 6

1. Ask the client to continue the Diary of Better Moments.
2. Ask the client to do the “Optimistic Thinking Style” exercise on a daily basis

Session 7

1. Ask the Opening Question About Progress "What's Better?"

Use the Diary of Better Moments.

2. Use EARS: Elicit, Amplify, Reinforce, Start Again

Invite the client to share positive information, then expand this information by asking questions about the details, and reinforce this positive information by being attentive and giving indirect compliments – for example, ask, "How were you able to do this?" or "How did you come up with that good idea?"

After highlighting the first example, ask again, "What else is better?" and continue asking "And what else?" Keep repeating the question, "What else?" to invite clients to look further than they might do initially. The most beautiful and important exceptions are often somewhat harder to find than the first and second answer.

Another often successful solution-focused question is this: First ask very pessimistic or depressed clients, "Please tell me about the worst moment since the last session." Listen respectfully and acknowledge the impact of the situation, but do not ask questions about details. Then continue, "So the other moments must have been at least a little bit better. Please tell me more about those."

3. Ask Scaling Questions About Progress

With scaling questions, therapists help clients to describe complex and intuitive observations of their past experiences and future possibilities. In this Session 6, use scaling questions to get a clear and concrete vision of their goal. Stick to a fixed order while searching for positive differences, starting with the question about the goal – the preferred future or preferred outcome

First, use scaling questions from 10 to 0, where 10 means the ideal situation, and 0 means the opposite. You do not have to ask any specific questions about 10 and 0: 10 just means all of their best hopes are met. Ask, "If 10 is the ideal situation, and 0 is the opposite, which number do you want to reach on that scale?" Their goal should be stated in realistic, concrete, and positive terms. Ask, "How exactly will your life be different?" and "What will you be doing differently?" inviting the client to give you a detailed description. Most clients will say that they want to reach a 7 or 8 on the scale.

The second question to ask is, "Where on the scale do you want your situation to be when you have finished this therapy?" The difference is the time perspective; the preferred future may be in a few years' time, but therapy is often shorter and therefore the feasibility of the goal might be different. You may start with a more general question, "Where do you want to end up on the scale?" and then ask, "Where on the scale do you want your situation to be at the end of therapy?" Or you may ask, "When can we stop meeting like this?" or "When is it not necessary to come here anymore?" Invite clients to give a detailed description of their preferred future from early in the morning until late

in the evening. What does their new and better life look like exactly? (Bannink, 2010, 2014, 2015a, 2015b).

The third question is, "What mark or number on the 10–0 scale do you give your current situation?"

Then, fourth, ask, "How is it that this number is not lower than it is?" "What is working?" "What else?" and "What else?" These questions focus on the exceptions and the client's competencies. Clients only need to do more of what works. This means that the solution does not have to come from you as their therapist!

The fifth set of questions is, "What does one point higher on the scale look like?" "How will you notice that your situation is one point higher?" "What will others notice that is different?" "How will they react (differently)?" "Who will be the least surprised?" "What will be next signs of progress?" or "Who will be the first to notice?"

Finally, the sixth question is, "Who or what may be useful to reach a higher number?"

Tip: Keep the triangle, *behavior–cognition–emotion,* in mind when inviting clients to describe their preferred future. Focus on positive differences compared with the present or the past, by always mentioning the term "different" or "differently":

Behavior: "What will you be doing differently?" (in the preferred future). Also use questions from other perspectives. "What will a friend see you doing differently, or family, or colleagues?" "How will they react differently?"

Cognitions: "How will you be thinking differently?" "How will you talk differently to yourself?"

Emotions: "How will you be feeling differently?"

4. Discuss the Homework Suggestions

Discuss the exercise "Optimistic Thinking Style."

5. Introduce the Concept of Gratitude

Explain the importance of *gratitude*. Say or read, "Research shows that people who are grateful are more cheerful, have more energy, and are less lonely. Researchers discovered that people who wrote a 'gratitude letter' to someone who has been important in their lives still felt happier 3 months later, than they did before they wrote the letter. Fredrickson (2009) found that gratitude is also good for your health. It appears that people who are grateful have fewer medical problems, a stronger immune system, and lower blood pressure."

Ask the client, "Which three people in your life have had a major positive influence on you? Who are they, and why were they important?" Reinforce and enhance what the client is saying, using EARS (Elicit, Amplify, Reinforce, Start again).

6. Do the Exercise "Gratitude in Four Steps" Together

Explain that this is an exercise to experience more gratitude in four steps. It allows you to experience more satisfaction and well-being." The four steps are as follows:

1. Focus on a few nongrateful thoughts – for example, the sun is shining, but I have to work all day.
2. Formulate grateful thoughts instead of those – for example, at least I have a job. Because I have a job, we live in a nice house, and we can go on holiday. Tomorrow the weather will be nice too, and I will have a day off. I also have a nice colleague with whom I collaborate well.
3. Replace the nongrateful thoughts with the grateful ones. Let the grateful thoughts really land, and pay attention to the feelings they produce. It may help to close your eyes for a moment.
4. Translate the positive feelings into action: Do something – for example, "I will get coffee for my colleague and tell her I am pleased to have her as a colleague. I am also going to invite my husband to go for a walk tomorrow morning."

7. Ask If the Client Wants to Do Some Homework Between This and the Next Session

If yes, then explain the homework suggestions (Homework Suggestions – Session 7).

8. Request the Client's Feedback, Using the SRS, and Ask the Follow-up Question

> Use the SRS, and then ask the follow-up question: What can I as a therapist do differently or better next time?

Homework Suggestions – Session 7

1. Ask the client to continue the Diary of Better Moments.
2. Ask the client to practice the exercise "Gratitude in Four Steps" on a daily basis.
3. Invite the client to write a Gratitude Letter.

Say to them:

> Close your eyes and recall the face of someone still alive who years ago did something or said something that changed your life for the better – someone you never properly thanked; someone you can meet face-to-face. Write a letter of gratitude to this person and deliver it in person. The letter should be concrete and about 300 words; be specific about what that person did for you and how it affected your life. Let this person know what you are now doing and mention how you often remember what they did. Once you have written the letter, call that person and tell them you would like to visit, but be vague about the purpose of your visit. This exercise is much more fun when it is a surprise.

When you meet the person, read the letter aloud to the recipient; take your time in reading the letter. Notice the reaction of the person listening to your words, as well as your own reaction. If the receiver interrupts you as you read, tell them you want them to listen until you are done. After you have read the letter (every word), discuss the content with the other person and share your feelings for each other.

If the person is no longer alive or lives too far away to actually visit, the gratitude visit may be adapted (e.g., make it imaginary or do it online).

Session 8

1. Ask the Opening Question About Progress "What's Better?"

Use the Diary of Better Moments.

2. Use EARS: Elicit, Amplify, Reinforce, Start Again

Invite the client to share positive information, then expand this information by asking questions about the details, and reinforce this positive information by being attentive and giving indirect compliments – for example, ask, "How were you able to do this?" or "How did you come up with that good idea?"

After highlighting the first example, ask again, "What else is better?" and continue asking "And what else?" Keep repeating the question, "What else?" to invite clients to look further than they might do initially. The most beautiful and important exceptions are often somewhat harder to find than the first and second answer.

Another often successful solution-focused question is this: First ask very pessimistic or depressed clients, "Please tell me about the worst moment since the last session." Listen respectfully and acknowledge the impact of the situation, but do not ask questions about details. Then continue, "So the other moments must have been at least a little bit better. Please tell me more about those."

3. Ask Scaling Questions About Progress

With scaling questions, therapists help clients to describe complex and intuitive observations of their past experiences and future possibilities. In this Session 6, use scaling questions to get a clear and concrete vision of their goal. Stick to a fixed order while searching for positive differences, starting with the question about the goal – the preferred future or preferred outcome.

First, use scaling questions from 10 to 0, where 10 means the ideal situation, and 0 means the opposite. You do not have to ask any specific questions about 10 and 0: 10 just means all of their best hopes are met. Ask, "If 10 is the ideal situation, and 0 is the opposite, which number do you want to reach on that scale?" Their goal should be stated in realistic, concrete, and positive terms. Ask, "How exactly will your life be different?" and "What will you be doing differently?" inviting the client to give you a detailed description. Most clients will say that they want to reach a 7 or 8 on the scale.

The second question to ask is, "Where on the scale do you want your situation to be when you have finished this therapy?" The difference is the time perspective; the preferred future may be in a few years' time, but therapy is often shorter and therefore the feasibility of the goal might be different. You may start with a more general question, "Where do you want to end up on the scale?" and then ask, "Where on the scale do you want your situation to be at the end of therapy?" Or you may ask, "When can we stop meeting like this?" or "When is it not necessary to come here anymore?" Invite clients to give a detailed description of their preferred future from early in the morning until late

in the evening. What does their new and better life look like exactly? (Bannink, 2010, 2014, 2015a, 2015b).

The third question is, "What mark or number on the 10–0 scale do you give your current situation?"

Then, fourth, ask, "How is it that this number is not lower than it is?" "What is working?" "What else?" and "What else?" These questions focus on the exceptions and the client's competencies. Clients only need to do more of what works. This means that the solution does not have to come from you as their therapist!

The fifth set of questions is, "What does one point higher on the scale look like?" "How will you notice that your situation is one point higher?" "What will others notice that is different?" "How will they react (differently)?" "Who will be the least surprised?" "What will be next signs of progress?" or "Who will be the first to notice?"

Finally, the sixth question is, "Who or what may be useful to reach a higher number?"

Tip: Keep the triangle, *behavior–cognition–emotion,* in mind when inviting clients to describe their preferred future. Focus on positive differences compared with the present or the past, by always mentioning the term "different" or "differently":

Behavior: "What will you be doing differently?" (in the preferred future). Also use questions from other perspectives. "What will a friend see you doing differently, or family, or colleagues?" "How will they react differently?"

Cognitions: "How will you be thinking differently?" "How will you talk differently to yourself?"

Emotions: "How will you be feeling differently?"

4. Discuss the Homework Suggestions

Discuss the exercise "Gratitude in Four Steps" and the Gratitude Letter. Also, as part of the Gratitude Letter, discuss the possible visit. Has the visit has already taken place, or is it still yet to happen?

5. Ask, Which Question(s) Have I Not Yet Asked That You Would Like to Hear?

Sometimes the therapist did not ask questions that the client deems important. In order not to overlook such questions, the therapist ask the client whether there are questions that they did not (yet) ask and the client would like to hear. Asking these questions may reveal important issues that did not come up during the sessions or were not addressed in a sufficient way.

6. Discuss the Usefulness of Continuing the Diary of Better Moments When Therapy Is Finished

It is important to keep a positive focus after the therapy has ended. Therefore, we invite you to continue to keep the Diary of Better Moments, to ensure that you stay focused on the exceptions to the problem and what you did to make that happen.

Earlier on we discussed that in these exceptions you can find what works in your life and what your competencies are. These are the things you can do more often in the future to create a new and better life.

7. Start Working on Behavior Maintenance During the Session; the Rest Will Be Part of the Last Homework Suggestion

Within positive CBT, we prefer to speak of *behavior maintenance* instead of *relapse prevention* (Bannink, 2012). Invite clients to find 50 things, in three different ways, for behavior maintenance:

1 Find 50 positive changes as a result of the therapy.
2. Find 50 good reasons to maintain those changes.
3. Find 50 ways to maintain those changes.

See Chapter 5 (The Case of Carin) for a few examples.

> Tip: Finding three times 50 things might seem a lot initially. Our tip: look for details. Everything counts – thoughts, behavior, feelings, posture, how you talk to yourself, what others have noticed, and so on. You may also include the third-person perspective, suggesting to the client, "Suppose I were to ask X (important other), what positive changes will they have noticed?" Clients may of course invite their loved ones to complete the list together with them.

8. This Time, Request the Client's Feedback for All Eight Sessions, Using the SRS, and Ask the Follow-up Question

> Use the SRS, and ask the follow-up question: What can I as a therapist do differently or better next time?

Homework Suggestions – Session 8

Complete the list of three times 50 things for behavior maintenance at home. Feedback from the therapist will no longer take place.

Chapter 4
Positive Cognitive Behavioral Therapy Protocol in a Group

The words you speak become the house you live in.

Hafiz, Persian poet

Introduction

In this chapter, we describe the positive CBT protocol for clients in a group, also in eight sessions. Fredrike drafted the first concept a few years ago in collaboration with colleague Fourough Jafari, who is affiliated with the Azad University of Tehran in Iran. Fredrike recently adjusted the protocol.

Positive CBT in a Group

The protocol for positive CBT in a group is based on Chapter 13 of *Practicing Positive CBT* (Bannink, 2012), which is titled "Positive CBT With Couples and Groups." In positive CBT in a group, the therapist works on strengthening the mutual cohesion in the group so that clients will assist each other and themselves in helping to find solutions for their issues. Clients are invited to contribute their experiences, ask each other questions, share things with each other, support each other, and make suggestions. This means no individual therapy is done in the group!

The exercises and discussion of homework suggestions are not always done with the group as a whole; clients work as much as possible in pairs and subgroups. It is the task of the therapist(s) to provide a pleasant atmosphere, safety, and a positive interaction process between the group members. It is their job to stimulate mutual conversations, involve everyone, and take care of those who need it.

Tips for positive CBT therapists working with a group:

- Don't do individual therapy in the group.
- Keep eye contact with all clients and pay attention to everyone.
- Invite clients to talk, respond, and help each other.
- Do not provide answers yourself, but ask clients to do so.
- Do not work on individual relationships; encourage mutual relationships instead.
- Do not start a conversation with individual clients; only stimulate conversations between them.
- Do not give your personal opinion.
- Find the personal strengths and resources of each client (VIA Character Strengths Survey, see Chapter 1).
- Look for resilience factors. These factors ensure that clients maintain a sense of well-being, even when adverse events occur. They are the psychological processes we use to address our strengths in adaptation to challenges (Bannink, 2014).

Brief Overview of Positive CBT Protocol in a Group

Below, you will find a brief overview of the positive CBT protocol in a group (Table 3). Each session lasts about 90–120 minutes; the number of clients can be up to eight people. One or two therapists may be present. When there are two therapists, they determine the division of tasks in mutual consultation beforehand.

Table 3 Brief overview of the positive CBT protocol in a group

Sessions	Activities	Homework suggestions
Session 1	1. Welcome and getting to know each other. 2. Building rapport with each client, "What do you do?" (work, study), "What are you good at?", and "What do you like about what you do?" 3. Invitation to design *group rules* (e.g., respect, tolerance, trust, confidentiality) 4. Explain rationale of positive CBT 5. Ask about *pretreatment change,* "What's already different or better since you first contacted us?" 6. Ask each client about their *goal.* "What will be the best result from this therapy for you?" or "What are your best hopes from this therapy?" and "What difference will it make when all your best hopes are met?"	1. *First session formula task:* observe daily what happens in your life that you want to keep happening (what does not need to change) 2. Exercise "Your Best Possible Self"

Table 3 continued

	7. Evaluate the collaborative relationship with each client 8. Explain the *first session formula task* and model this with one or two clients 9. *Positive imagination: "Your Best Possible Self"* – group exercise, enhancing optimism and hope 10. Memory support at the end of the session: "What do you take away from today?" 11. Require clients' feedback, using the GSRS	
Sessions 2–8	1. Ask each client, "What is better" (since the last time we met)? 2. Focus on exceptions: (small) successes and the clients' contribution to them) using EARS (De Jong & Berg, 2002) 3. Ask *scaling questions* to assess progress 4. Ask *competency questions,* "How did you do that?" and "How do you cope?" 5. Discuss the *take away* from the previous session (memory support) 6. Discuss clients' *feedback* and *homework suggestions* 7. Exercises during the session (see specific suggestions for each session). Do not do the exercise when clients do not want to do it, or when more time is needed to use EARS properly 8. Invite clients to start keeping a Diary of Better Moments (exceptions to the problem and/or the moments where already a glimpse is seen of their preferred future) 9. Ask clients if they find it useful to do certain homework suggestions. If yes, explain the suggestions and check if they have any questions 10. *Memory support*, "What do you take away from today's session?" 11. At the end of every session request *clients' feedback* using the GSRS (Duncan, 2010), including the question, "What can I (as your therapist) do better or different in the next session?"	

Table 3 continued

	All exercises and homework suggestions will now be discussed per session	
Session 2	1. Ask *scaling questions* about each client's goal. See to it that the goal from Session 1 is stated in positive, concrete, and realistic terms (also use results from exercise "Your Best Possible Self") 2. Invite clients to already think about *celebrating their successes*, "How are you going to celebrate your successes at the end of therapy when things are better?" 3. Explain importance of *finding exceptions:* keeping a Diary of Better Moments 4. *Find supporters* to help clients reach their goal 5. Introduce a *buddy system* in the group 6. Do exercise "Positive Gossip" (in groups of three or four) 7. Explain the VIA Character Strengths Survey	1. Buy a nice notebook or install a folder on your computer in which you keep your Diary of Better Moments 2. Write in your *Diary on a daily basis* 3. *Fill in the VIA Character Strengths Survey* online and bring it to the next session 4. *Find supporters* (family and/or friends)
Session 3	1. Exercise in subgroups, "What did you do so far today that is good for you?" 2. Demonstrate making a *topographic analysis*, based on their Diary of Better Moments, together with a couple of clients. Then also design a couple of positive FBA's with them, based on the same data. 3. Explain exercise "Three Blessings" and model with one or two clients 4. Discuss findings from the *VIA Character Strengths Survey* and how clients may use their top five to experience more well-being 5. Explain exercise "Positive Self-Portrait"	1. *Diary of Better Moments* 2. Daily exercise "Three Blessings" 3. Use *one of your signature strengths* on a daily basis 4. Start making a *Positive Self-Portrait* by interviewing five people. 5. Discussion will take place during Session 5, so no need to finish it before Session 4
Session 4	1. Exercise in subgroups: "Sparkling Moments" 2. Explain "Self-Compassion" – group exercise 3. Explain exercise "Letter From Your Future"	1. *Diary of Better Moments* 2. "Self-Compassion" exercise (daily) 3. Write a *Letter from your Future* 4. Finish your *Positive Self-Portrait*

Table 3 continued

Session 5	1. Ask, "What are you most proud of now you are halfway in therapy?" 2. Discuss their *Positive Self-Portrait* (homework started in Session 2) 3. Design more *topographical* and *FBAs* with clients based on their Diary of Better Moments 4. Explain finding "helpful beliefs and schemas" 5. Do exercise "Upward Arrow Technique" with some clients 6. Do exercise "Optimistic Thinking Style," with some clients (Seligman, 2002)	1. *Diary of Better Moments* 2. Exercise "Optimistic Thinking Style," on a daily basis
Session 6	1. Introduce "meaning." Ask clients, "What makes your life worth living?" and "Which five things do you do that contribute to a better world?" 2. Introduce "altruism" (Acts of kindness) 3. Explain the exercise "Acts of Kindness" 4. Group exercise: "Harmonica With Compliments" 5. Explain exercise "Gratitude in Four steps" – group exercise 6. Explain *Gratitude Letter*	1. *Diary of Better Moments* 2. Do five *Acts of kindness* per week all on one day 3. Exercise "Gratitude in Four Steps," on a daily basis 4. Write a *Gratitude Letter* and read the letter to that person
Session 7	1. Group exercise "Compliment Box" 2. Start discussing "behavior maintenance"	1. *Diary of Better Moments* 2. Three x 50 ways for *behavior maintenance* 3. Think about how you will *celebrate successes* in Session 8
Session 8	1. Read *compliments* from the box if there was no time to do so during Session 7 2. *Celebrate the clients' successes* with drinks and snacks 3. Make a *Certificate of Success* for each client (therapist and other clients together) 4. Memory support, "What do you take away from all 8 Sessions?"	1. Keep writing in your *Diary of Better Moments* 2. *Thank supporters* 3. *Thank your buddy* 4. Complete list of *Three x 50 things for behavior maintenance* at home 5. Set a *follow-up meeting* and notice what is going better in the meantime. Your therapist will ask about these better moments during the follow-up session

Follow-up session at 3–6 months	Follow-up session, live, or by Skype, email, or telephone. Session with the whole group or with each individual client. The opening question is, "What is better since the therapy ended?"	

Note. CBT = Cognitive Behavioral Therapy; EARS = Elicit, Amplify, Reinforce, Start again; FBA = Functional Behavioral Analyses; GSRS = Group Session Rating Scale.

For more detailed information about all exercises, please consult *Practicing Positive CBT* (Bannink, 2012). You will find more information and explanations about the exercises in the group protocol in the description of each session below (see Sections 4.4–4.11). In addition, you will find a comparison of the treatment protocols for individual positive CBT and positive CBT in a group at the end of this chapter (see Section 4.13).

Overview of the Sessions

Until recently, group therapy was usually done in a problem-focused way, and often individual therapy was done in the group. The aim was to reduce the individual problems of each group member. However, it is first and foremost the interaction between clients in a group that helps them to achieve their individual goals. Therefore, the goal of a positive CBT group is different: Its aim is to strengthen the group to assist the clients to help themselves and each other to find solutions to their personal issues and to build a better life. No individual therapy in the group is done. The group is responsible for contributing their experiences, questions, and willingness to share their experiences with each other, and to give support and suggestions. After all, they are all experts regarding their own life!

It is your responsibility as a therapist to ensure a pleasant and safe atmosphere and a positive interaction between the clients. It is also your task as a therapist to stimulate mutual conversation, involve everyone, and provide care to those who need it. Therefore, positive CBT in a group is not done *to* the group, but *with* the group.

Please note that if an exercise introduced in a session is used again in a later session, then we have repeated the instructions, but highlighted these with a thin black vertical line.

Ask the Opening Question About Progress, "What Is Better?"

The implicit suggestion of asking "What is better?" is *that* something is better, and clients only have to look at *what* it is that is better. Experience shows that if therapists always start with this opening question, clients are going to expect this question and will be able to come up with an answer sooner. If you, as their therapist, ask enough details about the past period, you will almost always find exceptions. These are the moments when the problem was expected to happen, but for some reason or another did not. These moments include when the problem was not there or was less (even just a little bit), and clients could cope better, and/or times when there were glimpses of the preferred future (their goal).

Note that the question, "What is better?" – in the present tense – is different from "How did things go last week?" or "What went well?" or even "What went better?" It initially requires some courage to be 100% predictable as a therapist using this specific opening question (which may be different from the question you used to ask). If there is no answer, you may ask, "So what is different?"

To find exceptions, please use the information from their Diary of Better Moments. Invite clients at the end of the second session and all subsequent sessions to write these exceptions down as a central homework suggestion. Say to them: "Please pay attention until the next session to the moments when things are a little better (or a little less bad), what you were doing differently then or were thinking or feeling differently, and what you did to make that happen. You will find the Diary of Better Moments in your Workbook (see Appendix 2)"

Use EARS: Elicit, Amplify, Reinforce and Start Again

By asking questions (elicit) invite clients to share positive information, expand it by asking questions about the details (amplify), and reinforce this by giving attention and indirect compliments (reinforce) – for example, ask, "How did you come up with that good idea?" After the first exception, you start again with "what else is better?" and then again, "And what else?" The question, "What else?" can be repeated often, inviting clients to search a little bit further than they would do normally. The most important exceptions are often a little further back on the shelf, so to speak, than the first and second answers.

Very pessimistic or depressed clients you may first invite to "tell me more about the worst moment of last week." Listen respectfully, and acknowledge their situation, but do not ask any questions about details. Then follow-up with "So the other moments must have been at least a little bit better, please tell me more about those."

Ask Competency Questions

During each session ask *competency questions*. Competency questions are a nice form of indirect compliments. They invite clients to tell a personal success story. Examples of competency questions are, "How did you do that?" "How did you decide to do that?" "How did you manage that?" "How did you come up with that good idea?" or "How do you cope?" The last question is a great one, especially for clients with whom you have a complainant relationship (clients who do not see themselves as part of the problem or solution; see Session 1, section 7).

Discuss the Clients' Feedback and Homework Suggestions

Invite clients to fill in the Group Session Rating Scale (GSRS). If there is still time left for feedback to be discussed, this can be done at the end of each session. If there is not enough time to discuss the feedback, do so at the start of the next session. At the end, always thank your clients for their effort and also ask, "What can I (as your therapist) do better or differently in the next session, so you will give a higher score at the end of that session?"

If clients give very high scores, you may ask a somewhat different question, “What should I continue to do in the next session, so that your score stays as high as it was at the end of this session?”

Always discuss the homework suggestions, and invite clients to share some examples of how they have dealt with things, with a clear focus on what went right instead of what went wrong.

In the following section we describe for each session all explanations, exercises, and homework suggestions belonging to that session, just like we did for the individual positive CBT protocol (Chapter 3). In Appendix 2, you will find the Client’s Workbook for Positive CBT in a Group. You can download the Client’s Workbook on the publisher’s webpage: Please see p. 144 for details.

Session 1

1. Welcome and Getting to Know Each Other

A warm welcome to the participants of the group. Introduction of the therapist(s) and all group members (see section 2.)

2. Building Rapport With Each Client

Warmly welcome all clients and invite them to share some information in response to the questions, "What do you do in your daily life?" (work, school, private), "What are you good at?" and "What do you like about the things you do?" The aim of these questions is to make the introduction a positive one, to build a positive collaborative relationship (rapport), and to get a positive image from the clients (who are always much more than the problems they suffer from). Such a positive introduction also serves as an icebreaker and indicates that this therapy might be different from what they expect, based on previous treatments or their ideas about psychotherapy.

3. Invitation to Design Group Rules

Clients should feel safe in a group. Therefore, invite them to determine the group rules themselves. Think of topics such as respect, tolerance, trust, and confidentiality.

> Tip: Ask clients to write the group rules on a flip chart and put the paper up in the therapy room during every session. It may be useful to briefly point out the rules now and again. Invite clients to do the same if necessary.

4. Explain the Rationale for Positive CBT

Share the following information with your clients (you can read it aloud, or say it in your own words):

> We will work with positive cognitive behavioral therapy – positive CBT. We will focus on your strengths and what works in your life – we are not focusing on what is wrong and what is not working. Focusing on your strengths and what works are the keys to start feeling better.
>
> We will also actively build on your well-being, positive thoughts, and positive feelings. They are important to experience more well-being. They are also a buffer against the impact of setbacks, and motivate us to explore our environment, make contact, and see and use opportunities. Research shows that people who suffer from depression experience fewer positive feelings. Moreover, it appears that for the recovery of depression the (re)creation of positive feelings, such as hope and gratitude, is more important than reducing negative feelings, such as fear and feeling sad. Research also shows that positive feelings protect us against relapse. Therefore, positive feelings are not only pleasant, but also important.

> We will also pay ample attention to what your preferred future looks like, to your personal strengths, and to the moments that are a little bit better or less bad. In addition, we will be watchful for those times when a glimpse of what you want to see instead of the problem (your preferred future) is visible. This is important, because these better moments (exceptions to the problem) are the keys to better functioning and more well-being – the keys to your better life.
>
> Positive CBT requires a different way of looking at things – you might say a different mindset. At first it may feel a bit strange if you have previously had psychotherapy that mainly looked at problems and how to repair them. In positive CBT, you certainly do not have to pretend there are no problems, or that you are not allowed to talk about them. However, we will focus first and foremost on what you would like to see, instead of the problems, and at which moments this is already the case, even just a little bit, and how you succeed in making this happen.

5. Ask About Pretreatment Change

Research shows that prior to the first session, two thirds of clients can give a positive answer to the question about *pretreatment change* (Weiner-Davis et al., 1987). Ask each client, "Many clients notice that in the time between making the appointment and the first session, things begin to improve already or are a bit better. What did you notice that is different about your situation during this time?" "What else did you notice?" and "What else?"

6. Ask Each Client About Their Goal (in Positive, Concrete, and Realistic Terms)

There are different ways to ask clients about their goal. You may ask, "What are your best hopes?" "What else are you hoping for?' "What difference will it make when all of your best hopes are met?" and "What difference will make it for important others?" Or you may ask, "What will be the best result of this therapy?" or "What do you want to see instead of the problem?"

Another way of defining the client's goal is to ask the *miracle question*: "Suppose a miracle happens while you are asleep tonight – the miracle being that tomorrow all problems are gone – but you didn't know because you were sleeping. What will be the first thing tomorrow morning that will tell you that this miracle has happened?" "What else will you notice that is different?" and "What else?" (NB: solution-focused questions are put in the unconditional future tense, so use "will," not "would.")

Also ask *scaling questions*, where 10 means the ideal situation, and 0 means the opposite. The order of asking scaling questions is as follows. First ask where on the scale the clients want their situation to be when they have reached their preferred future (or the end of therapy). Then, which mark on the scale do clients give their current situation, and how is it that it is not lower? Then, what does a higher mark look like? What will be different? And finally ask about how they could get there, "What and/or who may be useful in helping to get to a higher mark?"

7. Evaluate the Collaborative Relationship With Each Client With Regard to Their Goal

Do you have a visitor, complainant, or customer relationship with each client in the group? (NB: this is an estimate of the alliance between you as the therapist and each client; it is not a characteristic of the client!) This evaluation is important, because it offers a good indication of the client's motivation to change.

- Clients with whom you have a *visitor relationship* come involuntary; they are mandated (there is a referrer who thinks it is necessary for them to see you). Compliment them on their willingness to see you (at least once), and acknowledge the fact that they may be (somewhat) on the defensive side. Ask what they think the referrer wants to see to be different at the end of the therapy. Invite them to share their reactions and what they are willing to do. Do not give any homework suggestions.
- Clients with whom you have a *complainant relationship* come voluntarily, but do not see themselves as part of the problem and/or the solution: Someone else or something else needs to change. Acknowledge their suffering, and ask a specific set of solution-focused questions (Bannink, 2010, 2015b) to invite them to change themselves. Give only observational homework suggestions.
- Clients with whom you have a *customer relationship* also come voluntarily. They are the ones who do see themselves as part of the problem and/or solution. They are motivated to change and may receive both observational and behavioral homework suggestions. Remember: Ss long as you are not part of the solution, you are part of the problem!

This classification largely determines the course of the sessions and homework suggestions – for example, as a rule, clients with whom you have a complainant relationship need much more acknowledgment (a useful question being, "How do you cope with everything that is going on in your life?"), and only observational homework suggestions are suitable.

First ask clients (except clients with whom you have a visitor relationship) if they are willing to do some homework between sessions. If yes, explain each suggestion. Keep in mind that the central homework suggestion is keeping the Diary of Better Moments. If a client has not kept the diary for one reason or another, you may still ask about exceptions during the next session and emphasize the importance of looking at exceptions in positive CBT to find their competencies and what works in their lives. This may be done in front of the other participants, or may be done in pairs or trio's.

8. Explain the First Session Formula Task

Assume that there are always things in their lives that clients want to keep as they are or that should not change. Things that are going well (enough) which they might overlook, because they are so focused on what is not going well – for example, ask, "Between now and the next session please pay attention to what in your life you want to keep the way it is and what does not need to (or should not) change." This is an observational suggestion, so also suitable for clients with whom you have a complainant relationship. They only have to observe, not do anything different! This is called the *first session formula task*.

Invite clients "to pay attention between now and the next session when we meet, to everything in your life that you want to keep as it is or what should not change."

9. Explain the Exercise "Your Best Possible Self"

Research shows that "Your Best Possible Self" is a useful exercise for setting achievable and attractive goals, and increasing optimism and hope (Meevissen et al., 2011).

Say or read this to your clients:

> Imagine a moment in the future when you are at your best. Visualize your best possible self; a version of yourself that is very pleasing and which interests you. Imagine you have worked hard and succeeded in achieving your life goals. Think of dreams where you want to realize and use your own best potential. The point is not to think of unrealistic fantasies, but rather of things that are positive, attainable, and within reason.
>
> After you get a fairly clear image, write down the details. Writing down your thoughts and dreams helps to organize vague ideas and fragmented thoughts, so you can focus on concrete and real possibilities. Please write everything down in your Workbook and bring it to the next session.

10. Memory Support: "What Do You Take Away From Today?"

At the end of each session, ask each client, "What do you take away from today's session?" This can be done with the whole group or in subgroups. Research into memory support strategies shows that we remember only a little after having talked to a therapist or physician (Harvey et al., 2014). The researchers found that this does not only apply to patients with cancer or chronic pain, but also to clients with depression or a sleeping disorder (e.g., people with a sleeping disorder only remembered 13% of the session).

Harvey and colleagues developed eight strategies to improve memory recall in medical and psychological treatments. One of those strategies is applied in this protocol. At the end of each session ask, "What do you take away from this session?" Also, at the beginning of each subsequent session, you ask, "What did you take away from the previous session?" In every session, the therapist repeats these two questions and invites each client to share their thoughts. Everyone tends to remember different things, so clients can complement each other's memory.

11. Request the Clients' Feedback, Using the Group Session Rating Scale

Every time when using the GSRS, the follow-up question is, "What can I (as your therapist) and/or the group do differently or better the next session to get a higher score than today?" (see the Appendix in *Practicing Positive CBT,* Bannink, 2012; *Posttraumatic Success,* Bannink, 2014; and https:\\www.scottdmiller.com). If clients give very high scores, you may ask instead, "What should I and/or the group continue to do in order to receive the same high score, at the end of the next session, as you gave me and/or the group in this session?"

Homework Suggestions – Session 1

1. First session formula task: Between now and the next session, pay attention to what you want to keep in your life just as it is now, and what does not have to (or should not) change. Write this down in your Workbook.
2. Do the exercise "Your Best Possible Self."

Session 2

1. Ask Scaling Questions About Each Client's Goal

With scaling questions, therapists help clients to describe complex and intuitive observations of their past experiences and future possibilities. In Session 2, use scaling questions to get a clear and concrete vision of their goal. Add the findings from the exercise "Your Best Possible Self" to the description of their goal. With scaling questions, there is a fixed order, starting with the question about the goal – the preferred future or outcome.

First, use scaling questions from 10 to 0, where 10 means the ideal situation, and 0 means the opposite. You do not have to ask specific information about 10 and 0: 10 just means all of their best hopes are met. Ask, "If 10 is the ideal situation and 0 is the opposite, which number do you want your situation to be on that scale?" The goal should be stated in realistic, concrete, and positive terms. Ask, "How exactly will your life be different?" and "What will you be doing differently?" inviting clients to give you a detailed description. Most clients will say they want their situation in the future to be at 7 or 8.

The second question is, "Where on the scale do you want your situation to be when you have finished this therapy?" This is a different time perspective; the preferred future may be in a few years' time, but therapy is often shorter, and therefore the feasibility of the goal might be different. You may start with a more general question, "Where do you want your situation to end up on the scale?" and then ask, "Where on the scale do you want your situation to be at the end of therapy?"

You may also ask, "When can we stop meeting like this?" or "When is it not necessary to come here anymore?" Invite clients to give a detailed description of their preferred future from early in the morning until late in the evening. What does their new and better life look like exactly (Bannink, 2012, 2015b)?

The third question is, "What mark or number on the 10–0 scale do you give your current situation?"

Then, fourth, ask, "How is it not lower?" "What is working?" "What else?" and "What else?" These questions focus on the exceptions and the clients' competencies. Often clients only need to do more of what works. The good news is that the solution does not have to come from you as their therapist!

The fifth set of questions is, "What does one point higher on the scale look like?" or "How will you notice that your situation is one point higher?" "What will others notice that is different?" "How will they react (differently)?" "Who will be the least (the most?) surprised?" Or "What will be the next signs of progress?" or "Who will be the first to notice?"

And the sixth question is, "Who or what may be useful to reach a higher number?"

> Tip: Keep the triangle, *behavior–cognition–emotion,* in mind when inviting clients to describe their preferred future. Focus on positive differences compared with the present or the past, by always mentioning the term "different" or "differently":
>
> *Behavior:* "What will you be doing differently?" (in the preferred future). Also use questions from other perspectives, "What will a friend see you doing differently, or family, or colleagues?"
>
> *Cognitions:* "What will you be thinking differently?" or "How will you think differently of yourself?"
>
> *Emotions:* "How will you be feeling differently?"

2. Already Invite Clients to Think About How They Will Celebrate Their Successes

Ask each client, "How are you going to celebrate your successes when this therapy is over?" It is fun to do and useful (and often unexpected) to ask clients right at the start of therapy how they will celebrate their success. During the last session you can come back to this in detail. Celebrating successes, even small ones, motivates us to take next small steps.

3. Explain the Importance of Finding Exceptions

There are always exceptions if you and your clients are looking closely enough, even though they may think the problem is always there. After all, nothing stays the same; everything changes all the time. So it is not a matter of whether there are exceptions, but *when* they are happening.

Exceptions are those times when the problem could reasonably be expected, but for some reason or another did not occur. Ask clients the following questions (these all start with "when"):

- "When is or was the problem not there or is less (if only a little bit)?"
- "When is or was the problem not a problem?"
- "When is or was the problem there, but you succeed in coping a bit better?"
- "When is or was there a glimpse of your preferred future (you goal)?"

4. Find Supporters

Invite clients to select a few (two or three) supporters outside of therapy. It is easier to change when people support you, and you do not have to do it all by yourself. Those supporters can be family members, friends, or colleagues. Ask clients to explain to their supporters what their therapy goal is and discuss with their supporters how they can assist them in the best possible way. Ask clients to invite their supporters to explain to them why they trust that the clients can achieve their goal.

It is a given that clients will thank their supporters for their contribution at the end of therapy.

5. Introduce a Buddy System

Provide cards with two different colors. Half of the clients gets cards with one color, and the other half receive cards with the other color. Everyone writes their name on the card. The cards are folded and returned to the therapist (and perhaps placed in a box). Then ask everyone to choose a card other than their own color. Make sure no one sees who took which card. The person whose name is on the card drawn is to be their secret (or not so secret) buddy during the entire therapy. From that moment on, every client has a buddy and also functions as a buddy for another client in the group. Ask clients to make the life of their buddy as pleasant as possible.

When the group decides to keep the buddy a secret, clients may start to discover who might be their secret buddy, while their job is not to be unmasked. At the end of therapy, everyone guesses who their secret buddy was and thanks them. It is funny to see how clients sometimes guess the wrong person; the aim being to notice what acts of kindness people do for each other during therapy.

6. Do the Exercise "Positive Gossip"

Invite clients to do some "positive gossiping." Ask them to split up into groups of three (or four) people. Person A and B start positive gossiping for 2 minutes about person C, as if they were not there and could not hear them. Person C sits with their back to A and B and listens, but may not react.

After 2 minutes, the therapist gives a signal and clients switch roles: person B and C now gossip about person A for 2 minutes. Finally, person C and A gossip for 2 minutes about person B.

Clients always appreciate positive gossip. They like complimenting each other and often hear things about themselves that are new, moving, or amazing. Also, therapists often hear surprising (new) things that may change their ideas of their clients in a positive way!

7. Explain the VIA Character Strengths Survey

Invite clients to fill in the VIA Character Strengths Survey online (https://www.viacharacter.org/).

Explain that:

> everyone has certain strengths. By completing the questionnaire, you will discover your strengths, so you may increase them. Through this link you have to create an account first. Click ,on "Register," and then on "Continue" on the next screen. It takes about 30 minutes to complete the Survey; however, it is certainly worth it.

Tip: Please first fill in the Survey yourself as their therapist, if you have not done so already!

You may motivate clients by saying:

> It is very nice to see a list of your personal strengths; it often adds something to what you would say about yourself. Moreover, knowing your top five character strengths is important, because you can use them to enhance your well-being – engagement and meaning – and to experience flow.
>
> The outcome of the Survey will be sent to you via email. Bring the results of the Survey with you to the next session, so you can discuss the findings with your therapist and the other group members. It is also nice to hear about their top five and how they use these strengths in their lives!

8. Memory Support "What Do You Take Away From Today?"

As part of the memory support strategies, you, as their therapist, at the end of each session, invite the sharing of what everyone takes away from that specific session. At the beginning of each subsequent session, you also ask what they took away from the previous session.

9. Request the Clients' Feedback, Using the GSRS

Every time when using the GSRS, the follow-up question is, "What can I (as your therapist) and/or the group do differently or better the next session to get a higher score than today?" (see the Appendix in *Practicing Positive CBT*, Bannink, 2012; *Posttraumatic Success*, Bannink, 2014; and https:\\www.scottdmiller.com). If clients give very high scores, you may ask instead, "What should I and/or the group continue to do in order to receive the same high score, at the end of the next session, as you gave me and/or the group in this session?"

Homework Suggestions – Session 2

1. Invite the clients to keep a Diary of Better Moments throughout the therapy. Say to them, "Pay attention on a daily basis until the next session, to those moments in which things are a little bit better - or a little less bad - and notice what is different about those moments, and what you are doing differently at those moments."

Date	What happened?	What was better/ less bad?	What did I do differently?	What did I think/ feel differently?	What did I do to make that happen?

Tip: Also notice the moments which until now you may have overlooked. Also pay attention to the moments when things are just a little bit better or just a little less bad.

2. Complete the VIA Character Strengths Survey
   Complete the Survey online and bring the results to the next session.
3. Find supporters: Find two or three supporters (family, friends, or colleagues) who can assist you in making the desired changes. Explain what your goal in therapy is and how they may support you in reaching your goal. Note who your supporters are and how they are going to support you, in your Workbook.

Session 3

Start of Every Session

Ask each client in the group, "What is better" (since the last time we met)? Focus on exceptions: (small) successes and the clients' contribution to them, using EARS (Elicit, Amplify, Reinforce, Start Again).

Ask *scaling questions* to assess their progress and *competency questions,* "How did you do that?" "How did you cope?"

Discuss the take away from the previous session (memory support).

Discuss the clients' feedback from the last session and the homework suggestions they did since the last session.

1. Do the Exercise "Good for You"

This exercise can be done in a plenary session or in groups of two or three persons. We tend to pay more attention to what is not going well in our lives than to what is going well, "Bad is stronger than good" (Baumeister et al., 2001). To find a better balance, it is important to also look at what is going well. Therefore, invite clients to interview each other using these three questions:

1. "What have you done so far today that is good for you?"
2. "What else have you done so far today that is good for you?"
3. "And what else have you done so far today that is good for you?"

If clients cannot yet name three things, then ask,

1. "What will you do the rest of the day that is good for you?"
2. "What else will you do the rest of the day that is good for you?"
3. "And what else will you do the rest of the day that is good for you?"

2. Make Topographical Analyses and Positive Functional Behavior Analyses Together With Clients

Topographic analyses (TAs) are concrete examples of better moments, arising from the self-monitoring of exceptions. They serve as an aid for making positive *functional behavior analyses* (FBAs).

Positive FBAs of desired behavior or of better moments can be formulated in an ABC scheme, which refers to *antecedents* (situation), *behaviors and beliefs* (associated with desired or less undesired behavior), and *consequences* of the desired or less undesired behavior (positive – and if present – also negative effects). See Chapter 5 (The Case of Carin) for an example of a positive FBA.

Note that a negative C (consequence) is not obvious, but cannot be excluded either – for example, it may be that clients get less attention from the people around them when things are getting better.

3. Do the Exercise "Three Blessings"

Explain the exercise "Three Blessings" and do it with a couple of clients in the session. By way of setting an example the therapist demonstrates the exercise with a couple of clients in the session.

Research shows that doing this exercise even only for 1 week increases well-being immediately and continuously (it has been found to be noticeable 6 months later; Seligman, 2011). Many clients think it is a pleasant exercise and keep on doing it for longer than a week, but you do not really have to.

Say or read to the group, "Write down on a daily basis three good things that happened each day for a week. Those three things can be small (e.g., I went to bed early tonight, as I had planned) or large (e.g., the guy I've liked for months asked me out). Also write down what your part was in those good things and what they say about you."

4. Discuss the VIA Character Strengths Survey

Discuss the findings from their VIA Character Strengths Surveys during the session, especially their top five signature strengths, in plenary or in subgroups. Explain, "All 24 strengths are shown on the Survey. The order is important. The strengths at the top fit you best, the last ones the least. Therefore, do not dwell on the lowest strengths for too long, but focus on your own and each other's top five signature strengths instead."

As an alternative (if clients have not completed the Survey or have forgotten to bring the Survey), make a top five of their strengths as they see it, based on the list of 24 character strengths of Seligman and colleagues (see Table 2). Invite clients to choose three to five strengths and share some examples of how they applied these strengths lately. You may also use the third-person perspective (family, friends, colleagues). If clients cannot name anything or have little to say, suggest, "Suppose we were to ask your best friend(s) what they think your five strengths are, what do you think they would say?"

Every client has the same list of 24 character strengths, only in a different order of occurrence. It may happen that clients tend to focus on numbers 23 and 24 and think these should change. Do not dwell on those too long: Their top five is of signature strengths is far more important.

Also discuss how they can experience more *flow*. Flow refers to the mental state in which you are completely absorbed by your pursuits, such as making a painting or playing a musical instrument (Csikszentmihalyi, 1990). This is realized if there is an optimal balance between the difficulty of the task and the specific competencies you have. Furthermore, during flow, you can exceed your own skill level, learn faster, and gain new insights. Clients may experience more flow by using their top five signature strengths in a new area of life, or by deploying those strengths more often in an already existing area (e.g., work or hobby).

5. Explain the Exercise "Positive Self-Portrait"

Invite clients to:

> Ask at least five people who know you well to give you three written stories of instances when you did something positive in their life. If it is difficult to get written stories, it is also fine to receive them orally and write them down in your Workbook. But often a written story is the best thing.
>
> Collect all stories and read them to find common themes, surprises and insights. Summarize the stories as your Positive Self-Portrait and come up with a plan: How can you use your specific talents and strengths optimally? Then inform important people in your life about your plans.
>
> If you shy away from asking five (or more) people, it may help to reflect on the effect these conversations might have. You will get meaningful conversations with five (or more) people who are important to you; you will get positive reactions; you will probably get a valuable exchange about many domains of your personal and social life, work, spirituality, and so on. Think how valuable this may be for yourself, for important others and for your relationship with them.
>
> Please bring your Positive Self-Portrait to the fifth session. Take your time; you do not have to bring it to the next session, so you will have sufficient time to request positive feedback from important others.

6. Memory Support: "What Do You Take Away From Today?"

> As part of the memory support strategies, you, as their therapist, at the end of each session, invite the sharing of what everyone takes away from that specific session. At the beginning of each subsequent session, you also ask what they took away from the previous session.

7. Request the Clients' Feedback, Using the GSRS

> Every time when using the GSRS, the follow-up question is, "What can I (as your therapist) and/or the group do differently or better the next session to get a higher score than today?" (see the Appendix in *Practicing Positive CBT*, Bannink, 2012; *Posttraumatic Success*, Bannink, 2014; and https:\\www.scottdmiller.com). If clients give very high scores, you may ask instead, "What should I and/or the group continue to do in order to receive the same high score, at the end of the next session, as you gave me and/or the group in this session?"

Homework Suggestions – Session 3

1. Do the exercise Three Blessings: Say or read to the group, "Write down on a daily basis three good things that happened each day for a week. These three things can be small

(e.g., I went to bed early tonight, as I had planned) or large (e.g., the guy I've liked for months asked me out). Also write down what your share was in these good things and what they say about you."

2. Use one of your top five strengths on a daily basis: Say to the group, "You now know what your top five signature strengths are. Come up with a plan to utilize one of these strengths until the next session and then perform it daily. Write your choice of strength down in your Workbook and add exactly how you applied it and what the result was."
3. Start making your Positive Self-Portrait: Say to the group, "During the session I explained what a Positive Self-Portrait is about and how you can start making it. Please write everything down in your Workbook and bring it to the fifth session. Take your time, you don't have to bring it to the next session, but the one after that, Session 5."

Session 4

Start of Every Session

Ask each client in the group, "What is better" (since the last time we met)? Focus on exceptions: (small) successes and the clients' contribution to them, using EARS (Elicit, Amplify, Reinforce, Start Again).

Ask *scaling questions* to assess their progress and *competency questions,* "How did you do that?" "How did you cope?"

Discuss the take away from the previous session (memory support).

Discuss the clients' feedback from the last session and the homework suggestions they did since the last session.

1. Sparkling Moment

Invite clients to interview each other in groups of two or three about a recent *sparkling moment* in their lives:

1. "Think back to a (recent) moment in your life where you were at your best, a 'sparkling moment.'"
2. "Briefly describe that moment. What exactly did you do to make that moment sparkle?"
3. "What are you most pleased about?"
4. "Suppose others witnessed the sparkling moment, what will they have seen you doing?"
5. "If those competencies play an even greater role in your life, who will be the first to notice? What will they see you doing differently? What difference will that make?"

2. Introduce Self-Compassion

Introduce the concept of *self-compassion*. You don't necessarily have to use the term "self-compassion." Some clients may find that term too difficult or woolly. You may also refer to this as "being kind to yourself, even when you are struggling." Compassion is the ability to feel involved with pain and suffering, both our own suffering and that of others. Feeling compassion for others is usually easy, but feeling self-compassion is often much harder. Ask for exceptions, "When in your life did you succeed in having (a little) self-compassion?"

Do the "Self-Compassion" Exercise

Do this exercise together with the whole group.

Say to the group:

> "This is an exercise to be kinder to yourself. Think back to a recent moment when you were sad. Have you found one? Then please go back to that moment for a while. Experience the sadness again. Sit quietly, close your eyes, engage in your breathing, and then imagine yourself as a compassionate person. When you can feel that expanding and growing inside you, imagine you can see your own sad self in front of you. Look at their facial expression; note the feelings rushing through them. Just sit and feel compassion, and send compassionate feelings out to that sad self. Try to surround that sad self with compassion and understanding of the torment of sadness. For now, you are not trying to do anything other than experience compassion and acceptance. Imagine giving as much compassion and understanding as that sad part needs. You may want to imagine what happens to that sad part when it actually has all of the understanding and support it needs" (Gilbert, 2010, p. 171; in his exercise Gilbert uses anxietv instead of sadness).

If necessary, do the exercise twice, so clients are able to really feel it. You may also add a *soothing sign*. Invite clients to choose one themselves or ask them to put one hand on their shoulder. This is called cue conditioning and often has a positive effect. It is also possible to calm clients with words – for example, using a reassuring word or mantra, like "rest" or "relax."

3. Letter From Your Future

We humans are capable of *mental time travel*, forwards and backwards. That means that we can travel to the future or the past in our imagination, but also we can look back from the future to the present. That is exactly what we are going to do with this exercise.

Exercise: "Letter From Your Future"

Explain the exercise as follows:

> Write a letter from your future self to your current self (select a time that is relevant to you: 6 months, 1, 2, 5, or 10 years). Describe to yourself how well you are doing, include what you are doing, where you are, and so on. Also describe the crucial things you did to get there. And finally, give your current self some wise and compassionate advice from the future.

4. Memory Support: "What Do You Take Away From Today?"

> As part of the memory support strategies, you, as their therapist, at the end of each session, invite the sharing of what everyone takes away from that specific session. At the beginning of each subsequent session, you also ask what they took away from the previous session.

5. Request the Clients' Feedback, Using the GSRS

Every time when using the GSRS, the follow-up question is, "What can I (as your therapist) and/or the group do differently or better the next session to get a higher score than today?" (see the Appendix in *Practicing Positive CBT,* Bannink, 2012; *Posttraumatic Success,* Bannink, 2014; and https:\\www.scottdmiller.com). If clients give very high scores, you may ask instead, "What should I and/or the group continue to do in order to receive the same high score, at the end of the next session, as you gave me and/or the group in this session?"

Homework Suggestions – Session 4

1. Do the "Self-Compassion" exercise daily.
2. Write a Letter From Your Future.
3. Finish your Positive Self-Portrait: Describe your Positive Self-Portrait in your Workbook and bring it to the next session, even if it is not completely finished.

Session 5

Start of Every Session

Ask each client in the group, "What is better" (since the last time we met)? Focus on exceptions: (small) successes and the clients' contribution to them, using EARS (Elicit, Amplify, Reinforce, Start Again).

Ask *scaling questions* to assess their progress and *competency questions,* "How did you do that?" "How did you cope?"

Discuss the take away from the previous session (memory support).

Discuss the clients' feedback from the last session and the homework suggestions they did since the last session.

1. What Are You Most Proud of So Far?

At the start of the fifth session, the therapist asks each client what they are most proud of regarding their progress, now that they are halfway through therapy. The other clients are the verbal and nonverbal "cheerleaders": They give each other compliments on their achievements so far.

2. Discuss the Positive Self-Portrait

Most of the clients (all clients?) have now completed their Positive Self-Portrait. Invite them to discuss their Self-Portrait in subgroups of three or four people. The other clients are the cheerleaders.

Client:
These were really cheerful moments. That you believe, for the first time really start to believe, in yourself. The exercise of asking positive feedback from other people (Positive Self-Portrait) made clear that how I am beginning to see myself is now being confirmed by others.

I never realized that people see me the way they wrote about in their letters... positive, cheerful, taking initiative, you name it ... all very positive things. That realization is coming slowly during therapy. When it is confirmed by the people you love, it impresses more and has a greater effect.

3. Explain Finding Functional – Helpful – Thoughts and Beliefs

See Section 3.6: Session 3, Step 5, on how to design TAs and positive FBA.

Problems are the result of the client's perceptions about certain events (Bannink, 2012, 2017b). In addition to dysfunctional thoughts (cognitions) and (core) beliefs, we also have thoughts and beliefs which are the opposite of those. We call these our *functional* or *helpful* thoughts and beliefs.

Check with your clients to find which helpful thoughts and beliefs they have currently, and invite them to share some examples with you and the others. These helpful cognitions and beliefs do not have to be challenged (like dysfunctional or unhelpful cognitions and beliefs), because they are part of what works in the life of the client. Invite them to find out how these thoughts and beliefs are helpful and how they can use these more often than they already do.

Do the Exercise "Upward Arrow Technique"

By setting an example, the therapist demonstrates the exercise with a couple of clients.

Explain:

> Think of something in your life you would like to see changed for the better. Then ask yourself, "Suppose something in that situation improves, what difference will it make?" "What else will be different?" "What else?" "What will I be doing differently?" and "What else?" Discover that you can probably come up with more things than you first thought.

Other questions are, "Suppose it's possible for the situation to change, what will be different or better?" "What else?" "For yourself?" and "For others?" Or ask about the ***best-case scenario***, "What is the best that could happen?" "And suppose that does happen, what difference will that make?" as well as "And in its turn what difference will that make?"

The purpose of this exercise is to find out how many positive consequences one small change may generate. This exercise is often motivating and offers hope.

4. Introduce the Concept of Optimism

Explain the difference between pessimistic and optimistic thinking styles and their consequences.

Say or read:

> Pessimistic people attribute negative events, in particular, to stable, global and internal factors. They say, "Everything in my life is a mess" (stable), "I will never be happy again" (global), and "I am good for nothing" (internal). They attribute positive events to temporary, specific, and external factors. They say, "That was only luck; it had nothing to do with me" when something positive happens.
>
> Optimistic people tend to think the opposite way. They attribute positive events to stable, global, and internal factors. If something positive happens, they believe that it does say something about them – for example, 'I am a valuable person.' Optimists attribute negative events particularly to temporary, specific, and external factors. Thinking in a pessimistic way, especially about negative events, leads to hopelessness. The good news is that you can learn to be more optimistic and benefit from a more optimistic way of thinking.

Do the exercise "Optimistic Thinking Style" together with one or two clients. Say to them,

This is an exercise to become more optimistic:

- Every evening write a sentence in your Workbook about the best event of that day, as if it were caused by something stable, global, and internal (because I am ... or because I can ...) – for example, "Today a colleague offered to help me. This happened because I am someone who also helps others if needed."
- Every evening also write a sentence about the worst event of that day, as if it were caused by something temporary, specific, and outside yourself (because X, then Y) – for example, "Today I arrived late for my dentist appointment. This happened because the bus was delayed. This is the only time I have been late."

5. Memory Support: "What Do You Take Away From Today?"

As part of the memory support strategies, you, as their therapist, at the end of each session, invite the sharing of what everyone takes away from that specific session. At the beginning of each subsequent session, you also ask what they took away from the previous session.

6. Request the Clients' Feedback, Using the GSRS

Every time when using the GSRS, the follow-up question is, "What can I (as your therapist) and/or the group do differently or better the next session to get a higher score than today?" (see the Appendix in *Practicing Positive CBT*, Bannink, 2012; *Posttraumatic Success*, Bannink, 2014; and https:\\www.scottdmiller.com). If clients give very high scores, you may ask instead, "What should I and/or the group continue to do in order to receive the same high score, at the end of the next session, as you gave me and/or the group in this session?"

Homework Suggestions – Session 5

1. Do the exercise "Optimistic Thinking Style" on a daily basis, and write the sentences down in your Workbook.

Session 6

Start of Every Session

Ask each client in the group, "What is better" (since the last time we met)? Focus on exceptions: (small) successes and the clients' contribution to them, using EARS (Elicit, Amplify, Reinforce, Start Again).

Ask *scaling questions* to assess their progress and *competency questions,* "How did you do that?" "How did you cope?"

Discuss the take away from the previous session (memory support).

Discuss the clients' feedback from the last session and the homework suggestions they did since the last session.

1. Introduce the Concept of Meaning

Explain, "Giving meaning to your life is an important condition for well-being and resilience. Meaning can be found internally in our thoughts and reflections, and externally in our connection with others, charities and spirituality. Research shows that there is a strong positive relationship between meaning and psychological well-being" (Zika & Chamberlain, 1992). According to Viktor Frankl (1963), Holocaust survivor, life has meaning among all circumstances, even when there is unavoidable intense suffering. According to him, the challenge is to find meaning that is unique to each of us.

Life itself does not provide meaning, but it offers us the opportunity to determine what makes sense to us. Without a future perspective, making sense becomes more difficult, because what are you actually living for? A positive relation has been found between individuals who experience a lack of meaning and addictions (Crumbaugh, 1971).

Explain:

> A meaningful life is not just about yourself, but also about something higher or greater than yourself, a good cause and altruism: caring for others. Probably the higher or larger that other thing is, the more meaning we experience. It's about knowing what your top five signature strengths are (see the VIA Character Strengths Survey in Session 2) and putting those strengths at the service of something good, such as nature, or helping others.

Discuss with your clients in plenary or in subgroups during the session:

- What makes your life worth living?
- What five things do you do that contribute to a better world?

Afterwards ask clients to write down their answers in their Workbook.

2. Introduce the Concept of Altruism

Research shows that we will be happier through giving than we are through receiving. Introduce the concept of *altruism* (acts of kindness; Lyubomirsky, 2008): Do something nice for another person. See the exercise and homework suggestions for this session, on how to introduce and explain this in more detail.

3. Exercise: "Make a Harmonica With Compliments"

Ask each client to write their name on the top of a piece of paper (A4) and hand the paper to the person next to them. This person folds the paper, like a harmonica, and then writes a compliment to the person whose name is at the top of the paper. Then everyone hands the paper to the next person, after folding it again, so that the next person cannot read the previous compliment, but the name of the first person can still be seen. Eventually the paper returns to the person whose name is at the top, now full of compliments from all of the other clients. Surely, everyone keeps their paper!

4. Introduce the Concept of Gratitude

Explain the importance of gratitude:

> Research shows that people who are grateful are more cheerful, have more energy, and are less lonely. Researchers have discovered that people who wrote a Gratitude Letter to someone who has been important in their lives still felt happier 3 months later. Gratitude is also good for your health. It appears that people who are grateful have fewer medical problems, a stronger immune system, and lower blood pressure (Fredrickson, 2009). Gratitude is an important buffer against feeling depressed. When grateful, people focus on what they have instead of what thev don't have.

Do the Exercise "Gratitude in Four Steps"

By setting an example, the therapist demonstrates the exercise with a couple of clients.

Explain:

> This is an exercise to experience more gratitude in your life using four different steps. It allows you to experience more satisfaction and well-being. The four steps are:
> 1. Focus on a few nongrateful thoughts – for example, the sun is shining but I have to work today.
> 2. Formulate grateful thoughts instead of those – for example, at least I have a job. Because of this we live in a nice house and can go on holiday. Tomorrow the weather will be fine too, and I will have a day off. I also have a nice colleague with whom I collaborate well.
> 3. Replace the nongrateful thoughts with the grateful ones. Let the grateful thoughts really land and pay attention to the feelings they produce. It may help to close your eyes for a moment.
> 4. Translate the positive feelings into action: Do something – for example, "I will get coffee for my colleague and tell her I am pleased to have her as a colleague. I am also going to invite mv husband to go for a walk tomorrow morning."

"Gratitude Letter" Exercise

Invite clients to write a Gratitude Letter at home.

Say to them:

> Close your eyes and recall the face of someone still alive who years ago did something or said something that changed your life for the better – someone you never properly thanked; someone you can meet face-to-face. Write a letter of gratitude to this person and deliver it in person. The letter should be concrete and about 300 words; be specific about what that person did for you and how it affected your life. Let this person know what you are now doing and mention how you often remember what they did. Once you have written the testimonial, call that person and tell them you would like to visit, but be vague about the purpose of your visit. This exercise is much more fun when it is a surprise.
>
> When you meet the person, read the letter aloud to the recipient; take your time in reading the letter. Notice the reaction of the person listening to your words, as well as your own reaction. If the receiver interrupts you as you read, tell them you want Them to listen until you are done. After you have read the letter (every word), discuss the content with the other person and share your feelings for each other.

The Gratitude Letter can also be done in a virtual way. This may be of use if the person lives too far away to actually visit. If the person is deceased, the letter can be read out loud in their memory.

5. Memory Support: "What Do You Take Away From Today?"

As part of the memory support strategies, you, as their therapist, at the end of each session, invite the sharing of what everyone takes away from that specific session. At the beginning of each subsequent session, you also ask what they took away from the previous session.

6. Request the Clients' Feedback, Using the GSRS

> Every time when using the GSRS, the follow-up question is, "What can I (as your therapist) and/or the group do differently or better the next session to get a higher score than today?" (see the Appendix in *Practicing Positive CBT*, Bannink, 2012; *Posttraumatic Success*, Bannink, 2014; and https:\\www.scottdmiller.com). If clients give very high scores, you may ask instead, "What should I and/or the group continue to do in order to receive the same high score, at the end of the next session, as you gave me and/or the group in this session?"

Homework Suggestions – Session 6

1. Do the exercise "Acts of Kindness" (altruism): Introduce the exercise as follows: "Research shows that of all of the exercises which have been researched so far in the context of positive psychology, doing acts of kindness provides the most well-being. Do five acts of kindness all in one day (not one act a day, because then it may become boring and less effective). Do something that really makes a difference and requires some effort on your part, such as donating blood or helping your neighbors with their gardening, even if you do not really feel like it. Be creative and think about what people around you need the most. You may also turn the day in which you do the five acts of kindness into a ritual and insert a fixed day every week. Always find new acts of kindness which make a positive difference in the lives of others. After some time has passed, notice what difference this makes for others – and for yourself.
   "Do the exercise "Five Acts of Kindness" between now and the next session and notice what difference it makes for you and for others. Write down all acts of kindness in your Workbook.
2. Do the exercise "Gratitude in Four Steps" on a daily basis.
3. Write a Gratitude Letter and read it to that person.

Session 7

Start of Every Session

Ask each client in the group, "What is better" (since the last time we met)? Focus on exceptions: (small) successes and the clients' contribution to them, using EARS (Elicit, Amplify, Reinforce, Start Again).

Ask *scaling questions* to assess their progress and *competency questions,* "How did you do that?" "How did you cope?"

Discuss the take away from the previous session (memory support).

Discuss the clients' feedback from the last session and the homework suggestions they did since the last session.

1. Make a Compliment Box

Invite clients to make a *compliment box* during the session. First, they make or buy a beautiful box. During the session, each client puts a note with a compliment for each other client in the box. These notes are read aloud at the end of the session or if there has not been enough time to do so, during the eighth session. The compliments may be given anonymously or signed.

A variation of the compliment box is the *success box*. Each client is invited to anonymously submit three separate notes with solutions that have helped them successfully face or solve problems they experienced. Examples of solutions might be talking to a friend, taking long walks, or keeping a positive diary. When all the notes have been placed in the box, they are taken out and placed on a table. Each client can pick up one or two notes with solutions that are new to them (or which they want to try again), and try them out in a behavioral experiment, so in the next session they share with each other what worked and how it worked. In this way the expertise of the group is used optimally.

Think about whether you as their therapist would like to join or not. Or ask the group what they would prefer.

2. Start Working on Behavior Maintenance During the Session

In positive CBT, we prefer to speak of *behavior maintenance* instead of relapse prevention (Bannink, 2012, 2017b). We think it is more important to focus on keeping positive changes than to focus on preventing relapse. You may also do both.

Invite clients to start finding 50 things, three different ways, for behavior maintenance:

1. Find 50 positive changes as a result of therapy.
2. Find 50 good reasons to maintain those positive changes.
3. Find 50 ways to maintain those positive changes.

See Chapter 5 (The Case of Carin) for some examples and homework suggestions for this session. Completing the list is part of the homework suggestions for Section 4.12: Session 8.

3. Think About How You Will Celebrate Progress in Session 8

Think ahead and discuss with your clients how they will celebrate their progress during the last session. As their therapist, you may bring something tasty to eat and drink. Also, beforehand, design beautiful Certificates of Success (you will fill them in during the eighth session, together with the other clients).

4. Memory Support: "What Do You Take Away From Today?"

As part of the memory support strategies, you, as their therapist, at the end of each session, invite the sharing of what everyone takes away from that specific session. At the beginning of each subsequent session, you also ask what they took away from the previous session.

5. Request the Clients' Feedback, Using the GSRS

> Every time when using the GSRS, the follow-up question is, "What can I (as your therapist) and/or the group do differently or better the next session to get a higher score than today?" (see the Appendix in *Practicing Positive CBT*, Bannink, 2012; *Posttraumatic Success*, Bannink, 2014; and https:\\www.scottdmiller.com). If clients give very high scores, you may ask instead, "What should I and/or the group continue to do in order to receive the same high score, at the end of the next session, as you gave me and/or the group in this session?"

Homework Suggestions – Session 7

1. Start finding three times 50 things for behavior maintenance: Say to the group: "You probably achieved a lot in this therapy and made many positive changes. It is, of course, important to maintain these changes. During the last session, we began to do this. You are now invited to do the following:
   1. Find 50 positive changes as a result of therapy.
   2. Find 50 good reasons to hold onto these positive changes;
   3. Find 50 ways to maintain these positive changes.

Write everything down in your Workbook."

> Tip: Finding three times 50 things might seem a lot initially. Our tip? Look for details. Everything counts – thoughts, behavior, feelings, posture, how you talk to yourself, what others noticed, and so on. The clients may also include the perspectives of important others, such as their partner, children or friends. The therapist may suggest, "Suppose I were to ask them (important others), what positive changes would they say they had noticed?" Clients may of course invite their loved ones to complete the list together with them.

2. Determine how you will celebrate your successes: Say to the group, "During the second session, you have already discussed how to celebrate your successes at the end of therapy. That is exactly what we will do during the eighth session: We are going to celebrate what you and the others in the group have achieved. Everything counts, all small and big positive changes in your life. Think about how you would like to celebrate: Would you perhaps like to hang garlands, give a speech, thank your buddy, or bring a cake? Please inform me about your plans."

Session 8

Start of Every Session

Ask each client in the group, "What is better" (since the last time we met)? Focus on exceptions: (small) successes and the clients' contribution to them, using EARS (Elicit, Amplify, Reinforce, Start Again).

Ask *scaling questions* to assess their progress and *competency questions,* "How did you do that?" "How did you cope?"

Discuss the take away from the previous session (memory support).

Discuss the clients' feedback from the last session and the homework suggestions they did since the last session.

1. Discuss the Compliment Box (If Not Already Covered)

During the seventh session clients made a Compliment Box: Everyone has written a note with a compliment for the each of the other group members and placed it in the box. If there has been enough time to do so during the seventh session, the notes have already been read aloud. If not, the notes can be read now, at the start of this Session 8.

If the group chose the variation, the Success Box, those outcomes may also be discussed at this point.

2. Create a Certificate of Success

During this session, clients together with the therapist fill in a Certificate of Success (see Figure 4) for each group member (Bannink, 2014, 2015a). Nice formats for certificates can be found on the Internet. As their therapist, make sure the format for the certificates is ready at the start of this session. Design the Certificates in advance (but fill in the spaces indicated by dotted lines together with the other clients during this session).

3. Ask, "What Do You Take Away From the Entire Therapy?"

As part of the memory support strategies, you, as their therapist, at the end of each session, invite the sharing of what everyone takes away from that specific session. At the beginning of each subsequent session, you also ask what they took away from the previous session. Now you ask that same question, but this time it is about the entire therapy, not just Session 8.

4. Request the Clients' Feedback, Using the GSRS, This Time About the Whole Therapy

As with memory support strategies, invite clients to give their feedback again, but this time for all eight group sessions, the entire therapy.

Certificate of Success

We hereby state that

____

(name)

has successfully worked on

____

(goal)

This success was achieved by

____

____

____

____

____

(what worked)

____

Date

____

____

____

____

Signature
(name of therapist and other clients)

Figure 4 Certificate of Success

5. Schedule a Follow-Up Session

Schedule a follow-up session, in consultation with the group, after 3 or 6 months, with the group or with each individual client. The opening question, at this follow-up session, will be, "What is better since the therapy ended?" When scheduling the future session, the therapist informs the clients that that this will be the opening question.

Homework Suggestions – Session 8

1. Keep writing in the Dairy of Better Moments: Say to the clients, "Lately you have probably noticed how important it is to maintain a positive focus in your life. You probably feel better because of it and get a more positive perspective on yourself and the world around you. Although therapy has now ended, we recommend that you continue to fill in the Diary of Better Moments on a daily basis. It is a great way to keep on looking at the positive things that help you to achieve a better life."
2. Thank your supporters: Say to the group, "At the start of the therapy you invited a few people to be your supporters. We hope they supported you well. Now the time has come to thank them. Think about how you may do so. What do you think they would like? A nice greeting card, flowers, a big hug, a dinner? And then take action! Thank them from your heart."
3. Complete the list of three times 50 things for behavior maintenance: Say to the group: "In case you did not yet finish the list of three times 50 things for behavior maintenance, which you started during the previous session, please complete the list at home. Note: there is no longer feedback from the therapist and group members."

Comparison With the Protocol for Individual Therapy

In the treatment protocol of positive CBT in a group, our choice of exercises and homework suggestions has been somewhat arbitrary; many positive psychology exercises have proven to be effective, so we could have made other choices as well. You will find some of the same concepts and exercises in both protocols. F.B. has complied and adapted the group protocol more recently than the individual protocol. That is why you will find different points of focus in the group protocol from those in the individual treatment protocol.

Below are the highlights of the similarities between the individual and group protocol:

- A positive introduction and building *rapport*, with a focus on questions like, "What do you do?" "What are you good at?" and "What do you like about the things you do?"
- Explanation of the rationale of positive CBT.
- Questions about pretreatment change: positive changes prior to the first session.
- Goal formulation in positive, concrete, and realistic terms.
- Assessment of the collaborative relationship with regard to the goal.
- The question of whether clients find it useful to do certain exercises. The therapist should be flexible here.
- The request for feedback at the end of each session (in the individual treatment protocol with the SRS and in the group treatment protocol with the GSRS) and discussion at the beginning of each subsequent session (or when there is still time at the end of the same session). Asking the follow-up question, "What can I as your therapist do different or better in next session?"
- The homework suggestion at the end of the first session is the first session formula task: "What does not need to – or should not – change in your life?"
- The opening question about progress at the start of each subsequent session, "What is better?"
- The use of scaling questions about progress.
- Discussion of homework suggestions belonging to the previous session.
- The exercise "Your Best Possible Self," for further goal formulation – also a homework suggestion.
- The use of TAs and positive FBAs of exceptions.
- The use of scaling questions and competency questions.
- The Diary of Better Moments throughout the entire therapy.
- Completion of the VIA Character Strengths Survey and discussion of the findings.
- The exercise "Three Good Things" – also a homework suggestion.
- The "Self-Compassion" exercise – also a homework suggestion.
- The exercise "Upward Arrow Technique."
- The exercise "Optimistic Thinking Style" – also a homework suggestion.
- The exercise "Gratitude in Four Steps" – also a homework suggestion.
- The exercise "Five Acts of Kindness" – also a homework suggestion.
- The exercise "Positive Self-Portrait."
- Behavior maintenance: three times 50 things for behavior maintenance and completion of the list as the last homework suggestion.

Naturally there are also differences – for example, clients in the positive CBT group will design their own group rules during the first session. Furthermore, some exercises can only be done with more than one person. We highlight the following differences between the group protocol and individual protocol.

- In the group protocol, in the first session, clients design their own group rules (e.g., respect, tolerance, trust, confidentiality).
- Clients find a few supporters outside the group (family or friends) and a buddy within the group. Everyone becomes a buddy for another person and gets a buddy. The purpose of the buddy system is that the buddies take extra good care of each other during the sessions (and if desired also in between sessions).
- Clients use one of their signature strengths (their top five from the VIA Survey) on a daily basis.
- The therapist discusses functional – helpful – cognitions and beliefs with the group.
- The therapist discusses the concept of meaning and asks clients several questions about meaning.
- Clients write a Letter from their Future.
- Some exercises can only be done in a group and are therefore not applicable to individual therapy. These exercises are intended to enhance group cohesion and optimize their mutual expertise. These include the exercises involving the Harmonica of Compliments, Positive Gossip, Compliment Box, Sparkling Moment, and Good for You.
- In the group protocol, the exercise "Creating Powerful Beliefs" and the attendant homework are not included.
- In the second session of the group protocol, the therapist already asks how clients want to celebrate their successes at the end of therapy. In Session 7, they are invited to share their ideas on how they would like to celebrate the positive changes they have made, during the last session.
- At the start of the fifth session, the therapist invites each client to discuss what they are most proud of regarding their progress so far.
- At the end of each session, the therapist invites each client to indicate what they take away from the session. Also, at the start of each subsequent session, the therapist asks what they took away from the previous session. By inviting the clients to discuss this and think about it in an active way, it is more likely that they will remember more clearly what the session was about and what the most important things for them to take away are (the memory support strategies) (Harvey et al., 2014).
- During the eighth session, the clients celebrate their successes and thank their buddies in the group. The clients also thank their supporters when at home.
- During the eighth session, all clients receive a Certificate of Success made by the therapist and the other clients (Bannink, 2014, 2015a). On the beautifully designed Certificate the goal of the client is described and what the most important steps have been to bring that goal closer. Compliments from the therapist and other clients are added, as well as their signatures.
- A follow-up session is scheduled, after consultation with the group, for 3 or 6 months hence, with the entire group or with each individual client. The opening question will be, "What is better since the therapy ended?" The therapist makes it clear, when scheduling the session, that this question about progress will be the opening one.

Chapter 5
Case Carin

That you learn what being positive really is.
It was a steep learning curve for me because I couldn't do that.

Carin, client of positive CBT

Introduction

In this chapter, we describe a few excerpts from client Carin's individual positive CBT (fictitious name). We hope to paint a concrete picture of how positive CBT can look. She was one of the 49 clients who participated in the research protocol (see Chapter 2). Carin started with eight sessions of traditional CBT and then switched to eight sessions of positive CBT.

We describe only excerpts from the positive CBT process here.

Carin: Because I couldn't see things in a positive light, what the heck is seeing things positively? To understand that correctly and do something about it, you have to practice a lot before you realize: so this is how it works. That you learn what being positive really is.

It was a steep learning curve for me because I couldn't do that. I didn't know what love was and now I am finally learning to experience that.

Carin

Carin is a 22-year-old (or should we say young?) woman, who has been referred by her general practitioner. Since she was 15 years old, she has had recurrent depressive episodes. These episodes became longer and worse, and the current episode has been going on for more than 6 months. Carin never sought treatment before; she always tried to solve problems herself.

Carin describes herself as a "go-getter." She does not allow herself to show any weaknesses, and because of this, she often goes beyond her own boundaries. She has a tough attitude and gets angry and aggressive when she thinks other people do not understand her, or when they seem ungrateful. Inside, however, Carin says she feels sad and empty.

She has been living on her own for 2 years. Toward her parents she behaves in an adapted way; she often reluctantly does what her parents want her to do, instead of what she wants to do herself. In the intake interviews, borderline personality traits are suspected.

Goal Formulation and Scaling Questions

In Session 1, in addition to a positive introduction and building rapport, goal formulation takes place. As the best result from the therapy Carin wants to be able to give her life an 8 on a scale from 10 to 0. So what exactly does this 8 looks like? When she has reached an 8, she will be leading a positive life, will be pleased with herself, stand up for herself, and do what she likes to do (not what her parents want her to do), go out a lot, meet up with friends, and exercise regularly.

After eight sessions of traditional CBT, she rates her current situation as a 6 on the scale: She is starting to lead her life on her own terms, already pays more attention to her own needs, and is able to leave negative experiences behind more quickly by putting them into perspective. At the start of the traditional CBT sessions, she had rated her situation to be at a 4, and even rated it a 2 around the time of registration for therapy. When her therapist asked, "What will one mark higher on the scale look like?" – in other words, when Carin would rate her situation to be at a 7 instead of a 6 – she replied that then other people would see she was doing better. "What exactly will they see that is different? And what else will they see that is different?" asked the therapist. The answer to this was concretized during the session: Carin will be taking a more independent position, and will no longer be visiting her parents as often. Carin predicted that her parents would struggle with the fact that she would behave more independently (and no longer visit them three times a week). "I will have to explain it to them: This is how it works for me, how it is helping me. And I should be patient with my parents," she said.

What Is Better?

In Session 2, Carin completed the exercise "Your Best Possible Self." Elements of this are added to her previous goal formulation. Over time, Carin wants to have a loving relationship with a nice guy (not a "bad boy" – the type of guy she has fallen in love with in the past). Her Diary of Better Moments is also extensively discussed; the therapist reinforces this by paying a great deal of attention to these better moments and by giving many indirect compliments (in the form of competency questions).

Session 3 starts with the opening question, "What's better?" In between sessions, Carin told her mother that she will be visiting her less frequently. She managed to explain to her why she finds this important, she remained patient, and stood firm. And it worked out well: Although her mother was indeed disappointed, she was not angry and could understand her choice. Carin also had a good talk with her father, in which she revealed more about herself as a person. As a result, her father opened up a bit as well, and admitted that he found talking about his feelings difficult. Carin also made plans for attending a training course she had been interested in for a long time. At work she succeeded in standing up

<table>
<tr><th>Antecedent</th><th>Thoughts, behavior and emotion</th><th>Consequence</th></tr>
<tr><td>My parents want to see me more frequently than I want to see them.</td><td>Desired thoughts:
• I am a good person and daughter, even though I am not doing everything my parents want me to do.
Desired behavior:
• I am setting limits to my parents' claims on me.
Desired emotion:
• I feel calm, pleased with myself, proud.</td><td>Positive consequences:
• + c +: better mood (long term)
• + c +: more pleased with myself and proud (long term)
• + c +: better relationship with my parents (long term)
• – c –: less irritated by my parents (long term)
• – c –: fewer demands from my parents (long term)
• ~ c –: absence of self-blame (long term)
• ~ c –: absence of stress (long term)
Negative consequences:
• + c –: more claims from my parents (short term)
• + c –: more guilty feelings toward my parents (short term)</td></tr>
</table>

Figure 5 Positive functional behavioral analysis

for herself in a more capable way. She also received compliments from her colleagues. Together with her therapist, Carin makes a few topographical analyses (TAs) and positive functional behavioral analyses (positive FBAs), based on her self-monitoring of the better moments. In Figure 5, there is an example of such a positive FBA (see Figure 5).

"This Is What I Want"

To the usual opening question in the fourth session, "What is better?" Carin's replies, "Everything is just fine." Her mood is stable, and she is pleased with herself. She has made long working hours at her job. Carin and her therapist discuss her competencies. She did not fill in the VIA Character Strengths Survey, because she was not keen on spending half an hour sitting at her computer, but asked her family (as part of the exercise "Positive Self-Portrait") to write down a number of positive things about her. They replied that they think she is persistent and courageous, has integrity, and is honest and just. Carin is proud that she dared to ask her family to give her feedback. She also seized the opportunity to explain to her family how she wants her life to look in the future.

In the fifth session, Carin rated her current situation a 7, compared with her goal (a mark of 8 on the scale). Since she started positive CBT, she has put in more effort to explain to others exactly how she wants her life to look like. She stands up more for her own wishes. "I don't care so much anymore about what others think. This is what I want." By repeating this and explaining what she wants, she notices that she gets more appreciation and respect from other people.

The therapist asked her what some small, next steps or signs of progress might be, to reach an even higher mark on the scale. Carin replied, "Choose more situations myself, and be 'sincerely' happy with them. Be more patient with myself, and continue taking small steps forward and giving compliments to myself."

During the sixth session, Carin shared that she had done four acts of kindness, all in one day. It felt very positive, especially doing things for people other than her family. As an example, she helped her neighbor to retrieve his car from the garage. "It was nice to see how grateful he was." At work she indicated that she wants to work fewer hours. To reinforce her initiative, the therapist asked questions elaborating on the positive consequences of her decision. Advantages Carin identified are that she will have more energy as a result of more rest, will respond in a more positive way to her colleagues, which will be good for team spirit, and she will be 100% present mentally at work, which will be beneficial for her health in the long term. A disadvantage is that her boss will probably not like her decision of working less, because she will now need to find another solution for staff shortages. However, according to Carin, this disadvantage does not outweigh all of the benefits.

Together with the therapist, Carin does the exercise "Optimistic Thinking Style," in which successes are attributed to positive personal characteristics and her own commitment, while setbacks are attributed to external events and coincidences. Here is an example:

- *Most pleasant event of the day.* A colleague said "sorry" to me. This happened because I am very good at discussing their behavior, while also making clear that I am always there for them.
- *Most unpleasant event of the day.* My colleagues went to lunch without me. This happened because I came back a little later than usual and was not there when they departed.

Toward the end of the session, Carin indicated that she was doing very well and that she felt stable and strong. She wondered if she even still needed the remaining sessions. Because she was participating in the research protocol (and the quality of the research project benefitted from participants completing the full treatment), her therapist asked Carin whether she was willing to attend the two remaining sessions. Normally therapy could, at this point, be finished, because in positive CBT, the client is seen as coexpert, and decides when the therapy ends.

In the case of a decision by clients to end treatment, the therapist may ask scaling questions about their confidence to move forward on their own and their motivation to maintain the changes they made, and make a plan for behavior maintenance (see Session 8). However, Carin agreed to finish all eight sessions, especially because she liked them; the positive CBT sessions made her happy and gave her energy. This was in sharp contrast to her experience with the previous eight traditional CBT sessions with the same therapist, which she had found emotionally heavy and burdensome.

Gratitude

In the seventh session, Carin related that she had had a busy week at work and had seen many friends. Her mood had been stable, even often cheerful. In this session, the concept of gratitude was discussed. The therapist asked her which people in her life she was grateful for, and for what reasons.

One of her brothers plays an important role in her life; he is always there for her unconditionally. She is also grateful to have an older friend: He listens carefully, is empathetic, open, and clear. Carin was open to writing the two of them a Gratitude Letter (as a homework suggestion), but she did not want to read the letters to them. However, she did want to send the letters. The therapist reinforced the idea that Carin herself is in control of her life and able to make her own choices.

Also, the exercise "Gratitude in Four Steps," as a homework suggestion for the next week, was discussed during the session. Carin made the following statements:

Nongrateful thought: My father is not interested in me.

A grateful thought: My father does the best he can; sometimes he is a bit clumsy, and he is not good at sharing his feelings. But he is always there for me.

Replace the nongrateful thought with the grateful one.

Action: I am going to express gratitude to my father.

In answer to the therapist's scaling question how far Carin had progressed toward her goal (to reach a mark of 8), Carin gave her current situation a 7, and stated that this mark was very stable. "It takes time before I get to an 8, especially in relation to my parents. They are not able to show love, which often makes me feel undesired." The therapist asked how she wanted the relationship with her parents to be in the preferred future. And suppose her parents will not be able to show their love differently in the future, what can Carin herself do to improve the situation? She replied, "I am working on it. I should be patient, and repeat things over and over again. This takes time and does not change very quickly. I am trying to be more understanding. I am now confident that the situation slowly but surely will get better and better."

During the last session Carin felt completely relaxed. She had had a holiday and was reminiscing, "A wonderful feeling." During the last 2 weeks she had stopped doing specific exercises or recording homework suggestions. Relative to her goal (mark 8) she now gave her life a 7–7.5 and was happy with it.

Carin: It's about becoming more independent, discovering yourself, detaching yourself from your parents; that may take a while. It just needs time. If I keep up doing this until the end of the year, I think I will have made it.

Behavior Maintenance

Together with her therapist, Carin started completing the list of 50 positive changes, as part of her behavior maintenance plan. Here is a selection of the positive changes she made during therapy: She has more self-confidence, is more open, shares her feelings more since the last 2 months, does not always pretend to be tough, is exercising more, eats healthier food, is more relaxed, enjoys her life more, thinks first before she acts, has fewer conflicts, has stopped smoking, has lost 5 kg, has stopped seeing some "bad" people, has made better choices, is more patient, more confident, and more accepting.

Which 50 ways can Carin think of to maintain the positive changes she made? She already knows the following 12 ways: (1) keep talking to my parents and continue explaining how I want my life to be; (2) keep putting myself first more often; (3) buy time to make choices instead of responding immediately (e.g., by saying, "I first need to check my schedule"); (4) maintain a healthy lifestyle: exercising and not smoking (she had stopped smoking 2 months earlier); (5) visit my parents once a week, which is less than I did before; (6) continue to undertake activities with friends; (7) set aside moments for myself; (8) be more critical as to which persons I want to have as friends; (9) continue to show people that I am sometimes vulnerable; (10) keep my goal in mind; (11) keep thinking optimistically; and (12) continue to apply grateful thoughts instead of nongrateful ones.

Carin said she would finish the list at home. Of course, the therapist, being a "cheerleader," gave her a number of compliments on how far she had come.

Chapter 6
Frequently Asked Questions

The wisest person is not he who gives the right answers;
he is the one who asks the right questions.

Claude Levi-Strauss, French cultural anthropologist

Introduction

Below, you will find our answers to 12 frequently asked questions about positive *cognitive behavioral therapy* (positive CBT). In the many supervision hours during the research period for the participating therapists by CBT supervisor Fredrike, and in our training courses and presentations, these questions were often asked. We do not claim to give the only right answers and invite you to add your own answers to the list. There is no fixed order to the answers; you may try them all.

Twelve Frequently Asked Questions and Our Answers

Question 1: *What if my client cannot find a goal?*

- Ask what your client wants to have achieved by the end of the session(s).
- Ask what your client wants to see instead of the problem.
- Sometimes patients have never thought about their preferred future, so give them time to think about it, sleep on it, and/or discuss it with their loved ones.
- Give compliments for showing up and talking to you.
- Ask what the client's best hopes are and what difference it would make if all of their best hopes were met.
- Ask what they want to be better tomorrow, if the *miracle question* (see Chapter 3) does not provide sufficient information (e.g., in the case of autism).
- Invite the client to ask other people (e.g., family or friends) what they think their goal is.
- Ask for exceptions to the problem, when a glimpse of the preferred future is already present.

- Ask what is better or different since the signing up for the sessions (*pretreatment change*, see Chapter 3).
- Invite your client to do more of what works.
- Invite your client to pay attention to what works.
- Ask how your client is coping.
- Ask to exaggerate the problem (often they cannot).
- Ask about previous successes in solving problems to see what may be used again.
- Keep in mind that with your client you may not have a customer relationship and adjust your interventions accordingly.

Question 2: *What if the goal of my client is unrealistic?*
- If there is no solution, there is no problem (but a fact or disability). A problem can be solved; a fact or disability cannot be solved, and has to be dealt with in the best possible way (e.g., by accepting the fact or adjusting expectations). The focus is on possibilities instead of impossibilities.
- If your client has an unrealistic goal (winning the lottery, wanting someone who is deceased to be alive, wishing an accident never happened), ask, "Suppose that was a reality, what difference would that make in your life?" Or ask what this would mean to them.
- Ask yourself whether you are dealing with a complaint or wish (to bring about a different feeling or a change in another person) rather than an actual goal, the attainment of which lies within the client's control (in positive, realistic, and concrete terms).

Question 3: *What if my client cannot name any personal strength?*
- Help your client explore areas of their life that are going relatively well, expressing curiosity for their whole life, not just problem areas.
- Ask what is happening in their life that they wishes to keep as it is and link that to their strengths. Link these areas to the therapy goal.
- Ask coping questions and competency questions, "How do you manage?" "How do you cope?" and "How is the situation not worse?"
- Invite them to fill out the VIA Character Strengths Survey and discuss their top five signature strengths (see Chapter 1).
- Use the third-person perspective, "Suppose you had a twin brother or sister sitting right behind you (or a good friend), what would they say your personal strengths were?"

Question 4: *What if my client cannot find exceptions to the problem?*
- Do you have a complainant relationship with your client? (see Chapter 1). Then only give observational homework suggestions, such as, "What is going well and does not need to change?"
- Ask the client to observe the positive moments in their life so that they can talk about them the next time you meet.
- Ask them to pay attention to the times when things are going better (even just a little bit) so that they can talk about them the next time you meet.
- Invite your client to buy a beautiful notebook or install a folder on their computer and keep a Diary of Better Moments on a daily basis.
- Ask scaling questions:

> Where on the scale do you want your situation to be, when 10 means the ideal situation, and 0 the opposite? How exactly will your life look? Which mark do you give your current situation on that same scale? How is it not lower? What does a higher mark on the scale look like? What will you be doing differently? What will important people in your life say you will be doing differently? How will they react differently?

- Ask to pay attention to what gives them hope that the problem can be solved.
- Use prediction homework: "Predict what tomorrow will be like, find an explanation for why the day turned out the way it did tomorrow evening, and then make a new prediction for the following day."
- With a client in a complainant relationship, who thinks the other person is the problem and needs to change, say, "Pay attention to the times when the other person does more of what you want, what is different then, and pay attention to what they see you do then that is helpful to them in return."
- Ask the client to pay attention to what the other person does that is useful or pleasant and to the difference it makes, so that you can talk about it the next time you meet.
- Have them invite other people to tell them what exceptions they see.
- Ask, "Suppose you would find an exception, what difference will that make?"

Question 5: *What if my client says, "You tell me what to do, you are the expert!"*
- Ask your client if in the past it has been useful when other people told them what to do.
- Ask if, before you offer some suggestions, they would be willing to answer a few questions.
- Then, ask them about exceptions to the problem, their competencies and successes in the past.
- Keep them in the role of coexpert – for example, explain that others have solved problems similar to the client's problem through x, y, or z. Invite the client to reflect on which solution they may find most useful.
- Invite them to do some behavioral experiments and to observe what difference those make. For example, ask them to *pretend the miracle has happened* and observe the reactions of other people.
- Take a cautious stance, such as, "I think I have an idea, but I am sure you have already tried it and it probably didn't help much......did you ever try to....?"

Question 6: *What if my client comes up with an hypothesis or wants to find an explanation for what is wrong?*
- Remember that we humans are explanation seekers.
- Also remember that you do not need to find an explanation in order to be able to be useful for your client to reach their goal. Listen respectfully and go on with the conversation.

Steve de Shazer, cofounder of solution-focused brief therapy (SFBT), once commented on what you should do when you notice you are looking for a hypothesis or an explanation. He said, "Take two aspirins, go to bed and hope that it is over tomorrow" (de Shazer, personal communication). Because hypotheses limit one's view.

- Ask, "Suppose you would have an explanation, what difference will that make?"
- Ask, "How would an explanation be useful to you?"
- Ask, "What part of the explanation do you have already?"
- Ask what they can do to come up with information that may be useful in finding the explanation they want.
- Ask what explanations important others have come up with.
- The focus on hypotheses and explanations may indicate that you have a complainant relationship with this client (see Chapter 1).

Question 7: *What if my client has complex problems?*

- Remember that complex is not the same as difficult. It just means "compound or composite."
- Remember that complex problems do not need complex solutions and that you as a therapist do not need to know much about the client's problems to effectively be useful to them.
- Occam's razor, often expressed as the "law of parsimony," is a principle which recommends, when faced with competing hypotheses that are equal in other respects, to select the one that makes the simplest assumptions.
- Acknowledge the suffering from the problems the client has.
- Ask questions about the goal and exceptions, and ask scaling questions to invite the client to describe what they want to see differently and what mark they would give to their current situation on a scale from 10 to 0.
- Notice what type of working relationship you have with this client and attune your interventions and homework suggestions accordingly.
- Follow Einstein's constraint: Everything should be made as simple as possible, but no simpler.

Question 8: *What if my client has not done their homework?*

- Homework assignments as used in traditional psychotherapies (e.g., traditional CBT) are no longer seen as important in positive CBT. Change not only happens in between sessions, but also during the positive CBT sessions.
- Homework is only useful if the client finds it useful, so ask in advance if the client wants to do any homework. Only give behavioral suggestions when you have a customer relationship with this client.
- Ask yourself if homework will generate more information than if the client does not do any homework.
- Accept nonperformance as a message about your client's way of doing things rather than as a sign of resistance (see Chapter 3).
- Say that you are sure they must have a good reason for not doing the homework and invite them to tell you more about this reason. It is their way of showing the homework suggestion is not a good fit for them.
- If you see cooperation, you cannot see resistance; if you see resistance, you cannot see cooperation.
- Remember to keep a positive alliance, even without the client's having done any homework.

- Only provide feedback for the client to reflect on, or assign an observational homework suggestion instead of a behavioral one. You may not yet – or may no longer – have a customer relationship with this client (see Chapter 3).
- Do you want too much too soon? Look for small changes, use scaling questions regarding the client's goal, or counsel the client not to move too fast, and to take baby steps instead of big leaps.

Question 9: *What is the role of diagnostics in positive CBT?*

- The role of diagnostics is important, but diagnostics should not only be about problems, symptoms, disorders, and what is wrong in the client's life, but also about their personal strengths, resources, and what is going well. Discover the strengths of your client (e.g., by inviting them to fill in the VIA Character Strengths Survey) and what works in their life.
- Diagnostics should not only be about the problem (problem analysis), but also about what the client wants to see instead of the problem (goal formulation).
- The medical, problem-solving model assumes a necessary link between the problem and the solution. This assumption is reflected in the idea that problems must first be analyzed before solutions can be found. However, it is not (always) necessary to begin therapy with the mapping of problems.
- Analogous to stepped care, Bakker, Bannink, and Macdonald (2010) have presented their concept of *stepped diagnosis*. Ambulant intakes in primary or second-line health care are suitable for a solution-focused approach. During the first or follow-up session it will automatically become clear whether an advanced diagnosis will be necessary, for example if there is a visible deterioration in the patient's condition or if the treatment fails to give positive results. Analogous to *stepped care* one could think of *stepped diagnosis*.
- Diagnostics also concerns the nature of the alliance: Do you have a visitor, complainant, or customer relationship with your client? (see Chapter 1). This gives direction to your interventions and homework suggestions.
- In traditional CBT, self-monitoring, and functional behavioral analysis (FBA) are based on problems; in positive CBT, self-monitoring, and FBAs are based on exceptions to problems. For this reason, during the entire therapy, clients keep a Diary of Better Moments.

Question 10: *Are you never looking at the past in positive CBT?*

- Positive CBT is concerned with the past, but not to detect earlier problems and their causes. Rather it seeks to determine previous successes and competencies.
- Remember a past-present-future timeline is too simple an idea, and the present will also be shaped by how the future evolves (think of positive or negative *self-fulfilling prophecies*).
- Remember that the past is only the reminder in the present of past events and that the future is only our expectation in the present of later events. We only have access to the present.
- Positive CBT can change the meaning of what happened in the past. The (traumatic) past does not necessarily have to be discussed. When the present improves, and the patient gains more confidence in the future, the (traumatic) past will automatically become less toxic (Bannink, 2014, 2015b).

- Ask, "How will you know that what you have experienced will no longer stop you from living the life you want to live?" Or ask, "How will you know that you are doing justice to yourself and to your possibilities, in spite of what has happened to you?"
- See your clients as coexperts. "How did you succeed in shaping earlier changes in your life? Which competencies did you use? When were you able to use those strengths in other situations? Looking back, what makes it clear that you have always been able to do this?"
- Ask questions from the third-person perspective, "Who, of everyone you have ever known, would be the least surprised about those changes? Who would be the most surprised?"
- Ask the *miracle question*. Ask the client to imagine that the miracle has happened and their new and better life has begun, "When you look back what will tell you that you always knew you could do this?"

Question 11: *Is not positive CBT a bit problem-phobic?*
- In addition to discussing what works in their lives, clients are of course allowed to talk about problems; after all, positive CBT is not problem-phobic. As their therapist, you listen respectfully to their story and acknowledge their suffering.
- Clients often (still) think that talking about problems is the only form of psychotherapy available. Explain how positive CBT works and is different from traditional CBT or other problem-focused treatments. You may also give the client the choice between problem-focused and positive CBT.
- Positive CBT is not about solving clients' problems or complaints, but about the client's optimal functioning and their well-being.
- Reinforce *solution talk* instead of *problem talk*. Ask questions about the details of their preferred future, exceptions, and competencies. Do not ask questions about the details of the problem.
- Listen to the openings that always occur in every problem-saturated conversation and invite your client to describe what their new and better life looks like.

Question 12*: Does the relationship between the problem and solution get enough attention in positive CBT?*
- Einstein stated that you cannot solve problems with the same way of thinking with which they were created.
- There is not always a link between the problem and the solution, nor is it necessary to find one.
- The problem-solving model assumes that there is a necessary link between a problem and solution, using the medical model. This assumption is reflected in the idea that you must first have mapped the problem before solutions can be looked at. However, it is often not necessary to start therapy by mapping problems.
- The cause-and-effect medical model is applicable in cases of simply related, stable, and mechanical problems, but is not very useful in cases of complex and rapidly changing problems.
- Positive CBT does not rely on the cause-and-effect model (the *analysis paradigm*). It has been replaced by designing the preferred outcome (the goal; i.e., the *synthesis paradigm*).

You look forward to what might be created, rather than backward to how the problem came about and might be repaired.

- Some colleagues do not even use the term "solution," because it implies there is a problem. They prefer to speak of "designing an outcome" (De Bono, 1985) or possibilities and preferences (Walter & Peller, 2000).

Epilogue

The real voyage of discovery consists not in seeking new landscapes, but in having new eyes.

Marcel Proust, French writer

Through this book and the two treatment protocols, we want to make the application of *positive cognitive behavioral therapy* (positive CBT) easier and more pleasant for you. This approach will not only please your clients, as shown by our qualitative research, but it will be, as previous research also has shown, more pleasant for you as a therapist as well, and the positive focus may protect you from burnout (Medina & Beyebach, 2014).

Positive CBT offers the best constructive vision to date of what CBT can look like when joined with positive psychology and solution-focused brief therapy approaches. It offers a wealth of practical suggestions for how CBT therapists can become more positive in every aspect of therapy.

Christine Padesky, Center for Cognitive Therapy, USA

Proust stated that the landscape remains the same, but with new eyes a beautiful voyage of discovery is waiting for you!

References

Bakker, J. M., Bannink, F. P., & Macdonald, A. (2010). Solution-focused psychiatry. *The Psychiatrist, 34,* 297–300. https://doi.org/10.1192/pb.bp.109.025957

Bannink, F. P. (2010). *1001 Solution-focused questions: Handbook for solution-focused interviewing.* Norton.

Bannink, F. P. (2012). *Practicing positive CBT: From reducing distress to building success.* Wiley. https://doi.org/10.1002/9781118328941

Bannink, F. P. (2014). *Positieve cognitieve gedragstherapie* [Positive cognitive behavioral therapy]. Pearson

Bannink, F. P. (2014). *Post traumatic success: Positive psychology and solution-focused strategies to help clients survive and thrive.* Norton.

Bannink, F. P. (2015a). *Handbook of positive supervision.* Hogrefe.

Bannink, F. P. (2015b). *101 Solution-focused questions for help with Anxiety.* Norton.

Bannink, F. P. (2015c). *101 Solution-focused questions for help with Depression.* Norton.

Bannink, F. P. (2015d). *101 Solution-focused questions for help with Trauma.* Norton.

Bannink, F. P. (2017a). *201 Positive psychology applications.* Norton.

Bannink, F. P. (2017b). Positive CBT in practice. In C. Proctor (Ed.). *Positive psychology interventions in practice* (pp. 15–28). Springer. https://doi.org/10.1007/978-3-319-51787-2_2

Bannink, F. P. (2019). *Oplossingsgerichte vragen. Handboek oplossingsgerichte gespreksvoering* [Solution-focused questions. Handbook of Solution-focused conversations], 4th ed. Pearson

Bannink, F. P., & Peeters, F. (2020). *Practicing positive psychiatry.* Hogrefe.

Baumeister, R. F., Bratlavsky, E., Finkenauer, C., & Vohs, K. D. (2001). Bad is stronger than good. *Review of General Psychology, 5,* 323–370. https://doi.org/10.1037/1089-2680.5.4.323

Beck, J. S. (2011). *Cognitive behaviour therapy: Basics and beyond* (2nd ed.). Guilford Press.

Craske, M. G., Meuret, A. E., Ritz, T., Treanor, M., & Dour, H. J. (2016). Treatment for anhedonia: A neuroscience driven approach. *Depression and Anxiety, 33*(10), 927–938. https://doi.org/10.1002/da.22490

Craske, M. G., Meuret, A. E., Ritz, T., Treanor, M., Dour, H., & Rosenfield, D. (2019). Positive affect treatment for depression and anxiety: A randomized clinical trial for a core feature of anhedonia. *Journal of Consulting and Clinical Psychology, 87*(5), 457–471. https://doi.org/10.1037/ccp0000396

Crumbaugh, J. C. (1971). Frankl's logotherapy: A new orientation in counseling. *Journal of Religion and Health, 10,* 373–386. https://doi.org/10.1007/BF01532587

Csikszentmihalyi, M. (1990). *Flow: The psychology of optimal experience.* Harper & Row.

De Bono, E. (1985). *Conflicts, a better way to resolve them.* Penguin.

De Jong, P., & Berg, I. K. (2002). *Interviewing for solutions.* Brooks/Cole.

Demyttenaere, K., Donneau, A.-F., Albert, A., Ansseau, M., Constant, E., & van Heeringen, K. (2015). What is important in being cured from depression? Discordance between physicians and patients. *Journal of Affective Disorders, 174,* 390–396. https://doi.org/10.1016/j.jad.2014.12.004

De Shazer, S. (1985). *Keys to solution in brief therapy.* Norton.

De Shazer, S. (1991). *Putting difference to work.* Norton.

Duncan, B. L. (2010). *On becoming a better therapist.* American Psychological Association. https://doi.org/10.1037/12080-000

Duncan, B., Miller, S., Sparks, J., Claud, D., Reynolds, L., Brown, J., & Johnson, L. (2003). The Session Rating Scale: Preliminary psychometric properties of a "working" alliance measure. *Journal of Brief Therapy, 3,* 3–12.

Dunn, B. D. (2012). Helping depressed clients reconnect to positive emotion experience: Current insights and future directions. *Clinical Psychology and Psychotherapy, 19*(4), 326–340. https://doi.org/10.1002/cpp.1799

Dunn, B. D., Widnall, E., Reed, N., Owens, C., Campbell, J., & Kuyken, W. (2019). Bringing light into darkness: A multiple baseline mixed methods case series evaluation of Augmented Depression Therapy (ADepT). *Behaviour Research and Therapy, 120*(May), 103418. https://doi.org/10.1016/j.brat.2019.103418

Ferster, C. B. (1973). A functional analysis of depression. *American Psychologist, 28,* 857–870. https://doi.org/10.1037/h0035605

Frankl, V. E. (1963). *Man's search for meaning: An introduction to logotherapy*. Beacon Press.

Franklin, C., Trepper, T. S., Gingerich, W. J., & McCollum, E. E. (2012). *Solution-focused brief therapy: A handbook of evidence-based practice.* Oxford University Press.

Fredrickson, B. (2003). The value of positive emotions. *American Scientist, 91,* 330–335. https://doi.org/10.1511/2003.4.330

Fredrickson, B. (2009). *Positivity.* Crown.

Fredrickson, B. L., Mancuso, R. A., Branigan, C., & Tugade, M. M. (2000). The undoing effect of positive emotions. *Motivation and Emotion, 24*(4), 237–258. https://doi.org/10.1023/A:1010796329158

Garland, E. L., Fredrickson, B., Kring, A. M., Johnson, D. P., Meyer, P. S., & Penn, D. L. (2010). Upward spirals of positive emotions counter downward spirals of negativity. Insights from the broaden-and-build theory and affective neuroscience on the treatment of emotion dysfunctions and deficits in psychopathology. *Clinical Psychology Review, 30*(7), 849–864. https://doi.org/10.1016/j.cpr.2010.03.002

Geschwind, N. (2011). *From vulnerability to resilience against depression: The value of daily-life positive emotions* [Unpublished doctoral dissertation]. Maastricht University.

Geschwind, N., Arntz, A., Bannink, F., & Peeters, F. (2019). Positive cognitive behaviour therapy in the treatment of depression: A randomized order within-subject comparison with traditional cognitive behaviour therapy. *Behaviour Research and Therapy, 116,* 119–130.

Geschwind, N., Bosgraaf, E., Bannink, F., & Peeters, F. (2020). Positivity pays off: Clients' perspectives on positive compared with traditional cognitive behavioral therapy for depression. *Psychotherapy, 57*(3), 366–378. http://dx.doi.org/10.1037/pst0000288

Geschwind, N., Nicolson, N. A., Peeters, F., van Os, J., Barge-Schaapveld, D., & Wichers, M. (2011). Early improvement in positive rather than negative emotion predicts remission from depression after pharmacotherapy. *European Neuropsychopharmacology, 21*(3), 241–247. https://doi.org/10.1016/j.euroneuro.2010.11.004

Geschwind, N., Peeters, F., Jacobs, N., Delespaul, P., Derom, C., Thiery, E., & Wichers, M. C. (2010). Meeting risk with resilience: High daily life reward experience preserves mental health. *Acta Psychiatrica Scandinavica, 122*(2), 129–138. https://doi.org/10.1111/j.1600-0447.2009.01525.x

Gilbert, P. (2010). *Compassion focused therapy*. Routledge. https://doi.org/10.4324/9780203851197

Gotlib, I. H., Krasnoperova, E., Yue, D. N., & Joormann, J. (2004). Attentional biases for negative interpersonal stimuli in clinical depression. *Journal Abnormal Psychology, 113*(1), 121–135. https://doi.org/10.1037/0021-843X.113.1.121

Harvey, A. G., Lee, J., Williams, J., Hollon, S. D., Walker, M. P., Thompson, M. A., & Smith, R. (2014). Improving outcome of psychosocial treatments by enhancing memory and learning. *Perspective on Psychological Science, 9*(2), 161–179. https://doi.org/10.1177/1745691614521781

Hayes, S. C., Strosahl, K. D., & Wilson, K. G. (2003). *Acceptance and commitment therapy: An experiential approach to behaviour change.* Guilford Press.

Keyes, C. L. M. (2005). Mental illness and/or mental health? Investigating axioms of the complete state model of health. *Journal of Consulting and Clinical Psychology, 73,* 539–548. https://doi.org/10.1037/0022-006X.73.3.539

Khazanov, G. K., & Ruscio, A. M. (2016). Is low positive emotionality a specific risk factor for depression? A meta-analysis of longitudinal studies. *Psychological Bulletin, 142*(9), 991–1015. https://doi.org/10.1037/bul0000059

King, L. A. (2001). The health benefits of writing about life goals. *Personality and Social Psychology Bulletin, 27,* 798–807. https://doi.org/10.1177/0146167201277003

Kuyken, W., Padesky, C. A., & Dudley, R. (2009). *Collaborative case conceptualization.* Guilford Press.

Lyubomirsky, S. (2008). *The how of happiness.* Penguin.

Medina, A., & Beyebach, M. (2014). The impact of solution-focused training on professionals' beliefs, practices and burn-out of child protection workers in Tenerife Island. *Child Care in Practice, 20*(1), 7–36. https://doi.org/10.1080/13575279.2013.847058

Meevissen, Y., Peters, M., & Alberts, H. (2011). Become more optimistic by imagining a best possible self: Effects of a two week intervention. *Journal of Behavior Therapy and Experimental Psychiatry, 42,* 371–378. https://doi.org/10.1016/j.jbtep.2011.02.012

Peterson, C. (2006). The values in action (VIA) classification of strengths. In M. Csikszentmihalyi & I. Csikszentmihalyi (Eds.). *A life worth living: Contribution to positive psychology* (pp. 29–48). Oxford University Press.

Rashid, T. (2009). Positive intervention in clinical practice. *Journal of Clinical Psychology: In Session, 65*(5), 461–466. https://doi.org/10.1002/jclp.20588

Rush, A. J., Trivedi, M. H., Ibrahim, H. M., Carmody, T. J., Arnow, B., Klein, D. N., Markowitz, J. C., Ninan, P. T., Kornstein, S., Manber, R., Thase, M. E., Kocsis, J. H., & Keller, M. B. (2003). The 16-item Quick Inventory of Depressive Symptomatology (QIDS) Clinician Rating (QIDS-C) and Self- Report (QIDS-SR): A psychometric evaluation in patients with chronic major depression. *Biological Psychiatry, 54,* 573–583. https://doi.org/10.1037/t49873-000

Seligman, M. E. P. (2002). *Authentic happiness.* Free Press.

Seligman, M. E. P. (2005). Positive psychology, positive prevention and positive therapy. In C. R. Snyder & S. J. Lopez (Eds.). *Handbook of positive psychology* (pp. 3–10). Oxford University Press.

Seligman, M. E. P. (2011). *Flourish.* Free Press.

Seligman, M. E. P., Steen, T. A., Park, N., & Peterson, C. (2005). Positive psychology progress: Empirical validation of interventions. *American Psychologist, 60*(5), 410–421. https://doi.org/10.1037/0003-066X.60.5.410

Walter, J. L., & Peller, J. E. (2000). *Recreating brief therapy, preferences and possibilities.* Norton

Weiner-Davis, M., De Shazer, S., Gingerich, W. J., & Wallace, W. J. (1987). Building on pretreatment change to construct the therapeutic solution: An exploratory study. *Journal of Marital and Family Therapy, 13*(4), 359–363. https://doi.org/10.1111/j.1752-0606.1987.tb00717.x

Widnall, E., Price, A., Trompetter, H., & Dunn, B. D. (2020). Routine Cognitive Behavioural Therapy for Anxiety and Depression is More Effective at Repairing Symptoms of Psychopathology than Enhancing Wellbeing. *Cognitive Therapy and Research, 44*(1), 28–39. https://doi.org/10.1007/s10608-019-10041-y

Zika, S.. & Chamberlain, K. (1992). On the relation between meaning in life and psychological well-being. *British Journal of Psychology, 83,* 133–145. https://doi.org/10.1111/j.2044-8295.1992.tb02429.x

Zimmerman, M., Martinez, J. H., Attiullah, N., Friedman, M., Toba, C., Boerescu, D. A., & Ragheb, M. (2013). A new type of scale for determining remission from depression: The Remission from Depression Questionnaire. *Journal of Psychiatric Research, 47,* 78–82. https://doi.org/10.1016/j.jpsychires.2012.09.006

Zimmerman, M., McGlinchey, J. B., Posternak, M. A., Friedman, M., Atiullah, N., & Boerescu, D. (2006). How should remission from depression be defined: The depressed patient's perspective. *American Journal of Psychiatry, 163,* 148–150. https://doi.org/10.1176/appi.ajp.163.1.148

Appendix: Tools and Resources

For the therapist's convenience the appendices contain selected texts and informations for the client's workbooks.

Notes on Supplementary Materials

DOWNLOAD

The following materials for your book can be downloaded free of charge once you register on our website:

1. Client's Workbook for Positive CBT With Individuals
2. Client's Workbook for Positive CBT in a Group

How to proceed:

1. Create a user account (or, if you have already one, please log in)

For customers from the USA, Canada, and the rest of the world:
hgf.io/login-us

For European customers:
hgf.io/login-eu

2. Download your supplementary materials

Go to **My supplementary materials** in your account dashboard and enter the code below. You will automatically be redirected to the download area, where you can access and download the supplementary materials.

Code: B-KSCRJG

To make sure you have permanent direct access to all the materials, we recommend that you download them and save them on your computer.

Client's Workbook for Positive Cognitive Behavioral Therapy With Individuals

A warm welcome to you!

This is the Workbook which is aligned with your upcoming therapy. You do not have to read everything right now, you can do that later. Feel free to ask your therapist for help if needed.

Tip: Keep track of all of the exercises belonging to the homework suggestions. This way you will compile a useful reference book containing everything that works for you to feel mentally healthy(ier) and improve your well-being. Instead of using the worksheets, you could also buy a nice notebook or create a folder on your computer or phone.

What Is Positive Cognitive Behavioral Therapy?

Below is a brief explanation of what positive cognitive behavioral therapy (CBT) is exactly. You probably know that positive thoughts and feelings are important to feel better and experience more well-being. Positive thoughts and feelings form a buffer: They protect us against setbacks and motivate us to explore our surroundings, make contact, and see and use opportunities.

When we are depressed, we experience fewer positive feelings. Research has shown that experiencing more positive feelings such as hope, optimism, and gratitude is more important for recovery from depression than experiencing fewer negative feelings, such as fear and sadness. Positive feelings have also been found to protect against relapse and to decrease negative feelings.

In the next eight sessions, we will therefore focus on your well-being by promoting positive feelings and thoughts. We will also focus on what your preferred future looks like, look at your character strengths, and examine the moments when things go (a little bit) better or less bad in your life (exceptions to the problem).

This Workbook contains exercises that have been shown to improve our well-being. If you find it useful, you can do these exercises in between sessions. Your therapist will first discuss the exercises during the session, so that you will know exactly what to do.

We wish you lots of success and fun while participating in the positive CBT. We sincerely hope that this therapy will not only reduce your problems, but also increase your well-being. Please bring your Workbook to each session.

Client:
I really enjoyed the positive sessions. I looked forward to them every week. She [therapist] also stimulated my thinking, which was very nice. I think it is very difficult to change your thought pattern yourself. Especially in the beginning, I needed someone who invited me to see positive things in life. In the end, I managed to do this more and more by myself

Homework Suggestions – Session 1

Please keep track of all exercises and homework suggestions. You may also take notes of the sessions (the conversations you have with your therapist).

Exercise: "What Does Not Need to Change?"

We often only look at what needs to be changed or improved. That is understandable, but we often do not see things in our life that go well or well enough right now. Between now and the next session, please pay attention to everything that happens in your life (family, friends, work, relationships) that you want to keep happening or that should not change. Write these moments down in your Workbook and bring it to the second session.

Exercise: "Your Best Possible Self"

Your Best Possible Self is a future image about a new and better life. Imagine a moment in the future when you are at your best. Imagine Your Best Possible Self: someone you are particularly pleased with and who fascinates and interests you. Imagine that you have worked hard and succeeded in achieving your goal. Think of dreams that you want to realize using your specific talents. Your Best Possible Self is not about unfeasible fantasies, but about a positive and realistic goal. When you have a clear idea of what that is for you, consider the details and write them down.

Writing down these thoughts and what you dream of helps organize vague ideas and thoughts, so that they become concrete and achievable possibilities. Please write this exercise down in your Workbook and bring it to the next session.

Exercise: "Three Blessings"

As we mentioned at the start of this Workbook, we tend to look more often at what went wrong than at what went well. To find a better balance, record (at the end of each day, for 1 week) three good things that happened that day. Those three things can be small ("I went to bed early tonight, as I intended") or big ("The man I am in love with asked me for a date"). Also, write in your Workbook why those good things happened, what your influence was, and what they say about you. Please bring your Workbook to the next session.

Homework Suggestions – Session 2

Exercise: "Diary of Better Moments"

We often think that a problem is always present, but there are always exceptions if you look closely enough. Your therapist has already discussed this. Therefore, between now and the next session, pay attention every day to the moments when things go (a little bit) better or (a little) less badly. Those are the exceptions, which are always there, because nothing stays the same; everything changes. What exactly is different at those times? What do you do differently in those moments? What do you think and feel that is different then? What did you do to make that happen?

Fill in your Diary every day, and use the worksheets, where you have enough space to keep track of these Better Moments.

Date	What happened?	What was better/ less bad?	What did I do differently?	What did I think/ feel differently?	What did I do to make that happen?

Exercise: "(Start With) Your Positive Self-Portrait"

During the session, your therapist explained what a Positive Self-Portrait is and how to make it. Ask at least five people you know to give you three written stories of moments when you did something positive in their lives. If it is difficult to obtain written stories, you can also do this exercise verbally and then write the stories down in your Workbook – although its probably more fun to receive the written stories ...

Collect all the stories and read them again. What positive characteristics of yourself do you hear in their stories? Summarize the stories as your Positive Self-Portrait and write this down in your Workbook. Then come up with a plan: How can you best use your specific talents and strengths? Also inform important people in your life, such as your partner, children, or friends, about your plans.

If you are reluctant to ask five people (more than five is also allowed), it helps to reflect on the effect these conversations will probably have. You will have meaningful conversations with five people who are important to you; you will get positive reactions; you probably will have valuable conversations about many aspects of your personal and social life, work, spirituality, and so on. Consider how valuable this is to yourself, to others, and to your relationship with them.

Take your time; this does not have to be completed by the next session. Please bring your Positive Self-Portrait to the fourth session.

Homework Suggestions – Session 3

Continue the Diary of Better Moments

Between now and the next session, on a daily basis, pay attention to the times when things are (a little bit) better or (a little) less bad. What is different about those moments? What do you do differently in those moments? What do you think and feel that's different? What did you do to make that happen? Please write this down in your Workbook.

Fill in the VIA Character Strengths Survey

During the session your therapist explained what the VIA Character Strengths Survey is and how to complete it online. Everyone has certain strengths, and so do you. For the next session, complete the Survey online (https://www.viacharacter.org/). It takes about 30 minutes to complete the questionnaire, but it is well worth it. You get a list of all 24 strengths, including your top five signature strengths!

The order of the strengths is important: The strengths at the bottom say less about you, the strengths at the top say the most. So pay special attention to your personal top five. It is nice to see your strengths; the results from the questionnaire often help to add more to what you can say about your strengths. In addition, knowing your top five signature strengths is important: You can apply them to experience more well-being, engagement and meaning, and flow. Flow can be described as being fully immersed in a feeling of energized focus, full involvement, and enjoyment in the process of the activity.

The outcome of the Survey will be sent to you by email. Please bring the outcome of the Survey to the next session, so you can discuss this with your therapist.

Exercise: "Finish Your Positive Self-Portrait"

Finish your Positive Self-Portrait (from Sessions 2 and 3) and bring it with you to the next session, even if it is not yet completely finished.

Homework Suggestions – Session 4

Continue the Diary of Better Moments

Between now and the next session, on a daily basis, pay attention to the times when things are (a little bit) better or (a little) less bad. What is different about those moments? What do you do differently in those moments? What do you think and feel that's different? What did you do to make that happen? Please write this down in your Workbook.

Exercise: "Create Powerful Beliefs"

You will do this exercise with your therapist during the session. Between this and the next session, imagine the powerful beliefs on a daily basis, using Step 6: play the movie in your head.

1. What I would like to think about myself (desired belief)?
2. What would someone who has this belief naturally do (behaviors)?
3. In which future situation do I want to have this belief?
4. Choose behaviors from the list at Point 2 that show your desired belief and place yourself in that particular situation.
5. Imagine yourself in that situation while you behave in the desired way. Look at the situation, like a movie scene, in which "your future you" behaves in accordance with your desired belief. If useful, change the scene until it is positive and really fits.
6. Then return to the beginning of the scene. Step into the scene and experience it as if it is really happening. Look at everything and everyone around you, and notice how you feel. Hear how you express your belief with certainty. Go through the whole scene.

Homework Suggestions – Session 5

Continue the Diary of Better Moments

Between now and the next session, on a daily basis, pay attention to the times when things are (a little bit) better or (a little) less bad. What is different about those moments? What do you do differently in those moments? What do you think and feel that's different? What did you do to make that happen? Please write this down in your Workbook.

Exercise: "Self-Compassion"

During the session, your therapist discussed the concept of self-compassion: being kind to yourself. You may also describe self-compassion as thinking about yourself in a gentle way or feeling compassion for yourself. Think back to a recent moment when you were sad. Have you found one? Then please go back to that moment for a while. Experience the sadness again. Sit quietly, close your eyes, engage in your breathing, and then imagine yourself as a compassionate person. When you can feel that expanding and growing inside you, then imagine you can see your own sad self in front of you. Look at their facial expression; note the feelings rushing through them. Just sit and feel compassion, and send compassionate feelings out to that sad self. Try to surround that sad self with compassion and understanding of the torment of sadness. For now, you are not trying to do anything other than experience compassion and acceptance for your sadness. Imagine giving as much compassion and understanding as that sad part needs. You may want to imagine what happens to that sad part when it actually has all of the understanding and support it needs.

Exercise: "Five Acts of Kindness"

You will experience more happiness by giving than by receiving. Research has shown that, of all exercises that have been researched so far in the context of positive psychology, doing acts of kindness provides the most well-being. Do five acts of kindness all in 1 day (not one act a day, because then it may become boring and less effective). Do something that really makes a difference and requires some effort from your part, such as donating blood or helping your neighbors with their gardening, even if you do not really feel like it. Be creative and think about what people around you need the most. You may also turn the day on which you do the five acts of kindness into a ritual and insert a fixed day every week. Always find new acts of kindness that make a positive difference in the lives of others. Take some time to notice what difference this makes for others – and for yourself. Please write down all of your acts of kindness in your Workbook and bring it to the next session.

Homework Suggestions – Session 6

Continue the Diary of Better Moments

Between now and the next session, on a daily basis, pay attention to the times when things are (a little bit) better or (a little) less bad. What is different about those moments? What do you do differently in those moments? What do you think and feel that's different? What did you do to make that happen? Please write this down in your Workbook.

Exercise: "Optimistic Thinking Style"

You can actually learn to be more optimistic! Your therapist has already done this exercise with you during the last session. Now please do this exercise at home on a daily basis to train yourself to become more optimistic.

- Each evening, write down a sentence in your Workbook about the most pleasant event of that day, as if it were caused by something general (global), lasting (stable), and internal (because I am... or I can...).
  Example: Today a colleague offered to help me out. That happened because I am someone who also helps others when necessary.
- Each evening, also write a sentence about the most unpleasant event of that day, as if it were caused by something specific, temporary, and outside of yourself (because X then Y).
  Example: Today I arrived late for my dentist appointment. This happened because the bus had an unexpectedly large delay. This is the only time I have been late.

Below you will find another example of this exercise:

- Most pleasant event of that day. A colleague said "sorry" to me. This happened because I am very good at talking to people about their behavior, while also making clear that I am always there for them.
- Most unpleasant event of that day. My colleagues went to lunch without me. This happened because I came back a little later than usual, and they had already left.

Homework Suggestions – Session 7

Continue the Diary of Better Moments

Between now and the next session, on a daily basis, pay attention to the times when things are (a little bit) better or (a little) less bad. What is different about those moments? What do you do differently in those moments? What do you think and feel that's different? What did you do to make that happen? Please write this down in your Workbook.

Exercise: "Gratitude in Four Steps"

This exercise, designed so that you feel more gratitude, has four steps. It allows you to experience more satisfaction and well-being. You have already done this exercise with your therapist during the last session. Do this exercise on a daily basis until the next session and write down the four steps in your Workbook. The four steps are as follows:

1. Focus on a few nongrateful thoughts – for example, the sun is shining but I have to work all day.
2. Formulate grateful thoughts instead – for example, at least I have a job. Because I have a job, we live in a nice house, and we can go on holiday. Tomorrow the weather will be nice too, and I will have a day off. I also have a nice colleague with whom I collaborate well.
3. Replace the nongrateful thoughts with the grateful ones. Let the grateful thoughts really land and pay attention to the feelings they produce. It may help to close your eyes for a moment.
4. Translate the positive feelings into action: Do something – for example, I will get coffee for my colleague, and tell her I am pleased to have her as a colleague. I am also going to invite my husband to go for a walk tomorrow morning.

Exercise: "Gratitude Letter"

Your therapist has already discussed the Gratitude Letter. Close your eyes and recall the face of someone still alive who years ago did something or said something that changed your life for the better – someone you never properly thanked; someone you can meet face-to-face. Write a letter of gratitude to this person and deliver it in person. The letter should be concrete and about 300 words; be specific about what that person did for you and how it affected your life. Let this person know what you are now doing and mention how you often remember what they did. Once you have written the letter, call that person, and tell them you would like to visit, but be vague about the purpose of your visit. This exercise is much more fun when it is a surprise.

When you meet the person, read the letter aloud to the recipient; take your time in reading the letter. Notice the reaction of the person listening to your words, as well as your own reaction. If the receiver interrupts you as you read, tell them you want them to listen until you are done. After you have read the letter (every word), discuss the content with the other person and share your feelings for each other.

Include the Gratitude Letter in your Workbook. If the person is no longer alive or lives too far away to actually visit, you may adapt the gratitude visit to fit the situation (e.g., imaginary or online).

Homework Suggestions – Session 8

Continue the Diary of Better Moments

Between now and the next session, on a daily basis, pay attention to the times when things are (a little bit) better or (a little) less bad. What is different about those moments? What do you do differently in those moments? What do you think and feel that's different? What did you do to make that happen? Please write this down in your Workbook.

Exercise: "Make a Plan for Behavior Maintenance"

You probably have already achieved a lot in this therapy and made many positive changes. It is important to maintain those positive changes. We will start doing this during the last session. After the last session, continue to write items on the list of three times 50 things, and complete it. You can also ask important others in your life, such as your partner, children, or friends, to think along, or imagine what they would say if they were asked what positive changes you made – for example, "What would my partner say when asked what is going better?"

1. Find 50 positive changes as a result of the therapy.
2. Find 50 good reasons to maintain these positive changes.
3. Find 50 ways to maintain these positive changes.

Write everything down again in your Workbook.

> Tip: Finding three times 50 things might seem a lot initially. Our tip: Look for details. Everything counts – thoughts, behavior, feelings, posture, how you talk to yourself, what others have noticed, and so on.
>
> You may also include other perspectives, "Suppose I were to ask X or Y (important others), which positive changes would they have noticed?" You may invite your loved ones to help you to complete the list, if you wish.

Client's Workbook for Positive CBT in a Group

A warm welcome to you!

This Workbook accompanies your upcoming group therapy. The goal of the positive CBT group is to strengthen the group to assist you and the other group members to not only find solutions to the problems you are coming to therapy for, but also above all, to build a new and better life.

We would therefore like to invite you to contribute your own experiences, ask each other questions, share your stories, and offer each other support and suggestions. After all, you are the experts of your own life! Because of your expertise and the support you can give each other, group therapy may offer advantages over individual therapy.

The therapist will ensure that there is a positive and safe atmosphere and a positive interaction among you as participants. The therapist will encourage collaborative conversations, involves all of you and takes care of someone when needed.

This is the Client's Workbook for Positive CBT in a Group. You do not have to read everything right now, you can do that later. All exercises and homework suggestions will first be discussed in the group. Feel free to ask your therapist and/or other group members for help if needed.

Tip: Keep track of all exercises belonging to the homework suggestions. This way you will compile a useful reference book containing everything that works for you to feel mentally healthy(ier) and improve your well-being. Buy a nice paper notebook to write down your answers in, or create a folder on your computer or phone. Please bring this Workbook and your notes to each session.

What Is Positive Cognitive Behavioral Therapy?

We will start with a short explanation: What exactly is *positive cognitive behavioral therapy* (positive CBT)? During the next eight meetings (we call them sessions) this is what we are going to discover.

You probably know that positive thoughts and feelings are important to feel better and experience more well-being. Positive thoughts and feelings form a buffer: They protect us against setbacks and motivate us to explore our surroundings, make contact, and see and use opportunities.

Research has shown that when we are depressed, we experience fewer positive feelings. Experiencing more positive feelings, such as hope, optimism, and gratitude, has been found to be more important in recovering from depression than reducing negative feelings, such as fear and sadness. Positive feelings have also been found to protect against relapse and decrease negative feelings.

In the next eight sessions, we will therefore focus on your own and each other's well-being by promoting positive feelings and thoughts. We will also focus on what your preferred future looks like, look at your character strengths, and examine the moments when things go (a little bit) better or less bad in your life (exceptions to the problem).

This Workbook contains exercises that have been shown to improve our well-being. If you find it useful, you can do these exercises in between sessions. Your therapist will first discuss the exercises during the session, so you will know exactly what to do.

We wish you lots of success and fun while participating in the positive CBT. We sincerely hope that this therapy will not only reduce your problems, but also increase your well-being. Please bring your Workbook to each session.

> Client:
> I really enjoyed the positive sessions. I looked forward to them every week. She [therapist] also stimulated my thinking, which was very nice. I think it is very difficult to change your thought pattern yourself. Especially in the beginning, I needed someone who invited me to see positive things in life. In the end, I managed to do this more and more by myself.

Homework Suggestions – Session 1

Please keep track of all exercises and homework suggestions in your Workbook. You may also take notes during the sessions.

Exercise: "What Does not Need to Change?"

We often only look at what needs to change or improve. That is understandable, but we often do not see the things in our life that go well or go well enough right now. Between now and the next session, please pay attention to everything that happens in your life (in your family, friends, work, relationships) that you want to keep happening, or what should not change. Write these moments down in your Workbook and bring it to the second session.

> Tip: Consider also the small things you want to keep as they are. Maybe it is the kiss when your partner goes to work. Maybe it is the chat with your neighbor when you work in the garden. For inspiration, you can also ask people around you what they want to keep the way it is in their lives, and see if those things also apply to yours.

Exercise: "Your Best Possible Self"

Your Best Possible Self is a future image about a new and better life. Imagine a moment in the future when you are at your best. Imagine Your Best Possible Self: someone you are particularly pleased with and who fascinates and interests you. Imagine that you have worked hard and succeeded in achieving your goal. Think of dreams that you want to realize using your specific talents. Your Best Possible Self is not about unfeasible fantasies but about a positive and realistic goal. When you have a clear idea of what that is for you, consider the details and write them down.

Writing down these thoughts and what you dream of helps organize vague ideas and thoughts, so that you focus on concrete and achievable possibilities. Please write this down in your Workbook and bring it to the next session.

Homework Suggestions – Session 2

Exercise: "Diary of Better Moments"

We often think that a problem is always there, but there are always exceptions if only you look closely enough. Your therapist has already discussed this during the last session. Therefore, between now and the next session, please pay attention on a daily basis to the moments when things go (a little bit) better or (a little) less badly. Those are the exceptions, which are always there, because nothing stays the same; everything in this world changes. What exactly is different at those times? What exactly do you do differently in those moments? What exactly do you think and feel that is different then? What did you do to make that happen?

Fill in your diary every day, using your notebook, and bring your notes and this Workbook to the next session. We did not include extra space here, given that this is a daily exercise.

Date	What happened?	What was better/ less bad?	What did I do differently?	What did I think/ feel differently?	What did I do to make that happen?

Fill in the VIA Character Strengths Survey

During Session 2, your therapist explained what the VIA Character Strengths Survey is and how to complete it online. Everyone has certain personal strengths, and so do you. For the next session, complete the Survey online (https://www.viacharacter.org/). It takes about 30 minutes to complete the questionnaire, but this is well worth it. You will get a list of all 24 strengths, including your top five signature strengths!

The order of the strengths is important: The strengths at the bottom say less about you; the strengths at the top say the most. So pay special attention to your personal top five. It is nice to see your strengths; it often supplements what you can say about it yourself. In addition, knowing your top five signature strengths is important: When you apply them, you will experience more well-being, engagement, meaning, and flow. Flow can be described as being fully immersed in a feeling of energized focus, full involvement, and enjoyment in the process of the activity.

The outcome of the Survey will be sent to you by email. Please bring the outcome of the Survey to the next session, so you can discuss this with your therapist and other group members. It is also nice to hear about their top five strengths: how they apply those in their lives already and how they can use them even more often in the future!

Exercise: "Find Supporters"

Realizing a better life is easier if you do not have to do it alone, so think about who may be able to support you. Find two or three supporters (family members, friends, or colleagues) who can assist you in making the desired changes. Explain to them what your goal in therapy is: describe what you want to achieve. Also, explain how they can be useful. Perhaps they could occasionally ask how you are doing, or support you in completing certain homework suggestions. At the end of therapy, please thank your supporters for their support.

Note who your supporters are and how they are going to support you in your Workbook.

Homework Suggestions – Session 3

Continue the Diary of Better Moments

Between now and the next session, on a daily basis, pay attention to the times when things are (a little bit) better or (a little) less bad. What is different about those moments? What exactly do you do differently in those moments? What exactly do you think and feel that is different? What did you do to make that happen? Please write this down in your Workbook or on the worksheets.

Exercise: "Three Blessings"

As we mentioned before, we tend to look more often at what went wrong than at what went well. To find a better balance, at the end of each day, please record three good things that happened that day. Please do this exercise for 1 week. Those three things can be small

("I went to bed early tonight, as I intended") or big ("The man I am in love with asked me for a date"). Also write in your Workbook why those good things happened, what your influence was, and what they say about you. Please bring your Workbook to the next session.

Exercise: "Use One of Your Top Five Strengths on a Daily Basis"

By filling in the VIA Survey, you discovered your top five signature strengths. Read it again if you do not remember exactly what your top five are. The purpose of this exercise is to choose one strength on a daily basis and do something with it on that day - for example, suppose one of your strengths is curiosity. Then you could go and see a recent movie or visit a store that interests you and you have not visited yet. At the end of each day, write down in your Workbook what signature strength you used and what you did with it. It might be lots of fun!

Exercise: "(Start With) Your Positive Self-Portrait"

During the last session, your therapist explained what a Positive Self-Portrait is and how you can make it. Ask at least five people you know to give you three written stories of moments when you did something positive in their lives. If it is difficult to receive written stories, you can also ask people verbally and write their stories down in your Workbook (although written stories are the most fun to receive).

Collect all the stories and read them again. Which of your positive characteristics or strengths do you hear in their stories? Summarize the stories as your Positive Self-Portrait and write this down in your Workbook. Then come up with a plan: How can you make the best use of your specific talents and strengths? Also inform important people in your life, such as your partner, children, or friends, about your plans.

If you are reluctant to ask five people (more than five is of course allowed), it helps to reflect on the effect these conversations will probably have. You will have meaningful conversations with five people who are important to you; you will get positive reactions; you will probably have valuable conversations about many aspects of your personal and social life, work, spirituality, and so on. Consider how valuable this may be to yourself, to others, and to your relationship with them.

Please bring your Positive Self-portrait to the fifth session. Take your time; this exercise does not have to be completed by the next session.

Homework Suggestions – Session 4

Continue the Diary of Better Moments

Between now and the next session, on a daily basis pay attention to the times when things are (a little bit) better or (a little) less bad. What is different about those moments? What exactly do you do differently in those moments? What exactly do you think and feel that's different? What did you do to make that happen? Please write this down in your Workbook or on the worksheets.

Exercise: "Self-Compassion"

During the session, your therapist discussed the concept of self-compassion: being kind to yourself. You may also describe self-compassion as thinking about yourself in a gentle way. Feeling compassion for other people is often not so difficult, but many people find feeling compassion for themselves to be far more difficult. Do this exercise on a daily basis; it only takes a few minutes.

Think back to a recent moment when you were sad. Have you found one? Then please go back to that moment for a while. Experience the sadness again. Sit quietly, close your eyes, engage in your breathing, and then imagine yourself as a compassionate person. When you can feel that expanding and growing inside you, then imagine you can see your own sad self in front of you. Look at their facial expression; note the feelings rushing through them. Just sit and feel compassion, and send compassionate feelings out to that sad self. Try to surround that sad self with compassion and understanding of the torment of sadness. For now, you are not trying to do anything other than experience compassion and acceptance for your sadness. Imagine giving as much compassion and understanding as that sad part needs. You may want to imagine what happens to that sad part when it actually has all of the understanding and support it needs. You do not have to write things down here, just do the exercise.

Exercise: "Letter From Your Future"

Write a letter from your future self to your current self. Find a time that is relevant for you: 1, 2, 5, or 10 years in the future. Describe to yourself that you are doing well, explain what you are doing, where you are, and with whom. Also describe the main things you did to get there. What obstacles did you encounter and how did you overcome them? Finally, give your current self wise and compassionate advice from your future.

Exercise: "Finish Your Positive Self-Portrait"

Finish your Positive Self-Portrait and bring to the next session, even if it is not yet completely finished.

Homework Suggestions – Session 5

Continue the Diary of Better Moments

Between now and the next session, on a daily basis, pay attention to the times when things are (a little bit) better or (a little) less bad. What is different about those moments? What exactly do you do differently in those moments? What exactly do you think and feel that is different? What did you do to make that happen? Please write this down in your Workbook or on the worksheets.

Exercise: "Optimistic Thinking Style"

Optimism can be learned! Pessimistic people tend to attribute negative events to stable, global, and internal factors. They say, "Everything in my life is a mess" (stable), "I will never be happy again" (global), and "I am good for nothing" (internal). They tend to attribute positive events to temporary, specific, and external factors. They say, "That was only luck; it had nothing to do with me," when something positive happens.

Optimistic people tend to think the opposite way. They attribute positive events to stable, global and internal factors. If something positive happens, they believe that it does say something about them – for example, "I am a valuable person." Optimists attribute negative events to temporary, specific, and external factors. Thinking in a pessimistic way, especially about negative events, leads to hopelessness. The good news is that you can learn to be more optimistic and benefit from a more optimistic way of thinking.

You can actually learn to be more optimistic, even if you think you are a real pessimist! Your therapist has already done this exercise with you during the last session. Now please do this exercise at home on a daily basis to train yourself to become more optimistic.

- Each evening write down in your Workbook a sentence about the most pleasant event of that day, as if it were caused by something general (global), lasting (stable), and internal (because I am... or I can).
  Example: Today a colleague offered to help me out. That happened because I am someone who also helps others when necessary.
- Each evening also write a sentence about the most unpleasant event of that day, as if it were caused by something specific, temporary, and outside of yourself (because X then Y).
  Example: Today I arrived late for my dentist appointment. This happened because the bus had an unexpectedly large delay. This is the only time I have been late.
  Here is another example:
- Most pleasant event of that day. A colleague said "sorry" to me. This happened because I am very good at talking to people about their behavior, while also making clear that I am always there for them.
- Most unpleasant event of that day. My colleagues went to lunch without me. This happened because I came back a little later than usual and was not there when they left.

Homework Suggestions – Session 6

Continue the Diary of Better Moments

Between now and the next session, on a daily basis, pay attention to the times when things are (a little bit) better or (a little) less bad. What is different about those moments? What exactly do you do differently in those moments? What exactly do you think and feel that is different? What did you do to make that happen? Please write this down in your Workbook or on the worksheets.

Exercise: "Five Acts of Kindness"

Research has shown that we experience more happiness by giving than by receiving. Of all the exercises that have been researched so far in the context of positive psychology, doing acts of kindness provides the most well-being. Do five acts of kindness all in 1 day (not one act a day, because then it may become boring and less effective). Do something that really makes a difference and requires some effort from your part, such as donating blood or helping your neighbors with their gardening, even if you do not really feel like it. Be creative and think about what people around you need the most. You may also turn the day, on which you do the five acts of kindness, into a ritual and insert a fixed day every week. Always find new acts of kindness that make a positive difference in the lives of others. Take some time to notice what difference this makes for others – and for yourself. Please write down all your acts of kindness in your Workbook and bring it to the next session.

Exercise: "Gratitude in Four Steps"

Gratitude and grateful thoughts protect us from feeling sad and depressed. This is because, in thinking this way, you focus on what you have, instead of what you do not have. This is an exercise to enable you to experience more gratitude. It has four steps. It allows you to experience more satisfaction and well-being. You have already done this exercise with the other group members during the last session. Do this exercise on a daily basis until the next session and write down the four steps in your Workbook each day.

The four steps are as follows:

1. Focus on a few nongrateful thoughts – for example, the sun is shining, but I have to work all day.
2. Formulate grateful thoughts instead – for example, at least I have a job. Because I have a job, we live in a nice house, and we can go on holiday. Tomorrow the weather will be nice as well, and I will have a day off. I also have a nice colleague with whom I collaborate well.
3. Replace the nongrateful thoughts with the grateful ones. Let the grateful thoughts really land and pay attention to the feelings they produce. It may help to close your eyes for a moment.
4. Translate the positive feelings into action: Do something – for example, I will get coffee for my colleague and tell her I am pleased to have her as a colleague. I am also going to invite my husband to go for a walk tomorrow morning.

Exercise: "Gratitude Letter"

Your therapist has already discussed the Gratitude Letter. Close your eyes and recall the face of someone still alive who years ago did something or said something that changed your life for the better – someone you never properly thanked; someone you can meet face-to-face. Write a letter of gratitude to this person and deliver it in person. The letter should be concrete and about 300 words; be specific about what that person did for you and how it affected your life. Let this person know what you are now doing and mention how you often remember what they did. Once you have written the letter, call that person and tell them you would like to visit, but be vague about the purpose of your visit. This exercise is much more fun when it is a surprise.

When you meet the person, read the letter aloud to the recipient. Take your time in reading the letter. Notice the reaction of the person listening to your words, as well as your own reaction. If the receiver interrupts you as you read, tell them you want them to listen until you are done. After you have read the letter (every word), discuss the content with the other person and share your feelings for each other.

Include the Gratitude Letter in your Workbook. If the person is no longer alive or lives too far away to actually visit, you may adapt the gratitude visit (e.g., make imaginary or do it online).

Homework Suggestions – Session 7

Continue the Diary of Better Moments

Between now and the next session, on a daily basis, pay attention to the times when things are (a little bit) better or (a little) less bad. What is different about those moments? What exactly do you do differently in those moments? What exactly do you think and feel that is different? What did you do to make that happen? Please write this down in your Workbook or on the worksheets.

Exercise: "Make a Plan for Behavior Maintenance"

You probably already achieved a lot in this therapy and have made many positive changes. It is important to maintain those positive changes. We will start doing this exercise during the last session and then you will continue to write items on the list of three times 50 things and complete it.

1. Find 50 positive changes as a result of the therapy.
2. Find 50 good reasons to maintain these positive changes.
3. Find 50 ways to maintain these positive changes.

Write everything down again in your Workbook.

> Tip: Finding three times 50 things might seem a lot initially. Our tip: look for details. Everything counts – thoughts, behavior, feelings, posture, how you talk to yourself, what others have noticed, and so on.
>
> You may also include other perspectives, "Suppose I were to ask X or Y (important others), which positive changes would they say they have noticed?" You may invite your loved ones to help you to complete the list, if you wish.

Exercise: "Celebrating Successes"

In the second session, we already discussed how you would like to celebrate your successes at the end of therapy. In the last, the eighth, session we will celebrate all of the things you and your group members achieved. Everything counts, the very small and the big positive changes in your life. How would you like to celebrate your achievements? Would you like to hang up streamers, give a speech, thank your buddy, or bring a cake? Let your therapist know before the session starts!

Homework Suggestions – Session 8

Continue the Diary of Better Moments

Lately you have probably noticed the importance of maintaining a positive focus in your life. It makes you feel better and gives you a more positive view of yourself, the future, and the world around you.

Although the therapy is now over, we recommend that you continue to use the Diary of Better Moments on a daily basis. It is a good way to keep on looking at those things that help you get the better life you are looking for.

> Client:
> People should think more often about the things that are going well in their lives, and that is exactly what this therapy is about. I noticed that if you focus on the things that are going well, the things that are not going well will automatically fade into the background.

Exercise: "Thank Your Supporters"

At the start of this therapy you invited a few people to be your supporters. We hope they were of help to you. Now the time has come to thank them. Think about how you might do so: What do you think they will appreciate? A greeting card, flowers, a big kiss, a dinner? And then take action! Thank them from your heart.

Exercise: "Complete the List of Three Times 50 Behavior Maintenance"

In case you did not finish the list of three times 50 things for behavior maintenance, which you started during the previous session, please complete the list at home. Note: there is no longer feedback from the therapist and other group members.

Follow-up Appointment

During the last session, your therapist discussed with you and other group members when and how a follow-up session will take place. For your information: the therapist's opening question will be, "What is better since the therapy ended?"

Acknowledgments

It is often said that an author never writes a book alone. It is always the product of many people working together, even though only the names of the author(s) appear on the cover.

First of all, I want to thank my coauthor Nicole Geschwind. It was her idea to start a study of positive CBT and to develop the protocol for individual positive CBT for this purpose. I am pleased with her great enthusiasm for this treatment approach and our pleasant collaboration in recent years.

I thank my Iranian colleague Fourough Jafari for sharing her ideas for the positive CBT group protocol.

I also thank all my clients, colleagues, students, and teachers for their inspiration: because of them I still enjoy my work very much.

I thank my husband, Hidde, for his unconditional love and support: He is always there for me. And finally, once again, *mille grazie* to my four Italian cats, who kept me company during the many supervision hours conducted on Skype and during the writing of this book.

Fredrike Bannink

I would like to thank Fredrike Bannink for our inspiring collaboration. During my PhD project about resilience against depression, I discovered the importance of positive emotions for mental health. I started looking for ways to better stimulate and use positive emotions in the treatment of psychopathology. At a CBT conference I attended a presentation by Fredrike and immediately became enthusiastic about positive CBT. We decided to set up a research project together to investigate the effectiveness of positive CBT as a treatment approach for depression. That is now 6 years, a training course, and many supervision sessions ago.

I also want to thank my colleagues, friends, parents, and in-laws for all the inspiration, support, and fun moments.

And, of course, I thank my three tough, but very sweet men: Sibren, Jamie, and Ando; I love you!

Nicole Geschwind

Together we thank Arnoud Arntz and Frenk Peeters for the pleasant collaboration and their contribution to our research. We thank Arnoud for his comments on an earlier version of this book. We also thank Emke Bosgraaf for conducting the interviews and his important role in our qualitative research. We thank the therapists Cristel Achterberg, Nienke Jabben, and Patrick Fokkema for their openness to applying this approach in CBT, which was also new to them and sometimes felt a bit uncomfortable. We also thank all clients for their courage and willingness to collaborate with our research.

We thank our colleague Suzanne Aldis Routh in Toronto for her scrutinous supervision of the English translation. We are sure her work made our translation a better one.

Finally, we would like to thank all employees of Hogrefe Publishers for their contribution to the realization of this book. We are very pleased to welcome the English translation of our book, which was originally published in Dutch in 2019.

Fredrike Bannink and Nicole Geschwind

About the Authors

Fredrike Bannink is a clinical psychologist, child psychologist, and lawyer. She is a trainer and supervisor of the Dutch Association for Behavioral and Cognitive Therapies (VGCT) and cofounder and chair of the Positive CBT section. She is also founder and chair of the Special Interest Group (SIG) Positive CBT of the European Association for Behavioural and Cognitive Therapies (EABCT).

Her interests lie in the fields of positive psychology and solution-focused interviewing. She is an international keynote speaker, trainer, and author of about 50 books (https://www.fredrikebannink.com).

Nicole Geschwind is an assistant professor at the Department of Clinical Psychological Science at Maastricht University. Her research interests are in the field of resilience to depression, in particular the value of positive emotions. By systematically examining the role of positive emotions in facilitating change, and by testing the benefits of a stronger focus on positive emotions in clinical settings, she hopes to contribute to improving psychotherapy.

Notes on Supplementary Materials

DOWNLOAD

The following materials for your book can be downloaded free of charge once you register on our website:

1. Client's Workbook for Positive CBT With Individuals
2. Client's Workbook for Positive CBT in a Group

How to proceed:

1. Create a user account (or, if you have already one, please log in)

For customers from the USA, Canada, and the rest of the world:
hgf.io/login-us

For European customers:
hgf.io/login-eu

2. Download your supplementary materials

Go to **My supplementary materials** in your account dashboard and enter the code below. You will automatically be redirected to the download area, where you can access and download the supplementary materials.

Code: B-KSCRJG

To make sure you have permanent direct access to all the materials, we recommend that you download them and save them on your computer.